Understanding Alzheimer's
Disease and Other Dementias

of related interest

The Simplicity of Dementia
A Guide for Family and Carers
Huub Buijssen
ISBN 978 1 84310 321 9
eISBN 978 1 84642 096 2

Dementia – Support for Family and Friends
Dave Pulsford and Rachel Thompson
ISBN 978 1 84905 243 6
eISBN 978 0 85700 504 5

Hearing the Person with Dementia
Person-Centred Approaches to Communication for Families and Caregivers
Bernie McCarthy
ISBN 978 1 84905 186 6
eISBN 978 0 85700 499 4

Can I tell you about Dementia?
A guide for family, friends and carers
Jude Welton
Illustrated by Jane Telford
ISBN 978 1 84905 297 9
eISBN 978 0 85700 634 9

Understanding Alzheimer's Disease and Other Dementias

Brian Draper

Jessica Kingsley *Publishers*
London and Philadelphia

First published in Australia in 2011 by Longueville Media

This edition published in 2013 by Jessica Kingsley Publishers
116 Pentonville Road
London N1 9JB, UK
and
400 Market Street, Suite 400
Philadelphia, PA 19106, USA

www.jkp.com

Library of Congress Cataloging in Publication Data
Draper, Brian.
 Understanding alzheimer's disease and other dementias / Brian Draper.
  pages cm
 Includes bibliographical references and index.
 ISBN 978-1-84905-374-7 (alk. paper)
 1. Alzheimer's disease. 2. Dementia. I. Title.
 RC523.D73 2013
 616.8'31--dc23
                             2013005842

British Library Cataloguing in Publication Data
A CIP catalogue record for this book is available from the British Library

ISBN 978 1 84905 374 7
eISBN 978 0 85700 883 1

Printed and bound in Great Britain by Bell & Bain Ltd, Glasgow

Contents

Acknowledgements

I have had a lot of support from my family in writing this book with my wife Debbie giving very sensible advice on the text and my daughters Leah and Sally providing encouragement.

I would like to acknowledge Professors Colin Masters, Brian Lawlor and Simon Lovestone for their expert opinions that I canvassed for Chapter 13 in the first edition of this book, and Professors Gary Small, David Ames, Perminder Sachdev, Henry Brodaty and Michael Woodward for their expert opinions that I canvassed for Chapter 13 in both the first edition and this current edition.

Preface

Alzheimer's disease is well established in the community as being a major cause of memory impairment and progressive, usually irreversible, mental decline in old age, otherwise known as dementia. While there are many other conditions that can cause dementia, Alzheimer's disease is the most common and attracts the greatest attention – so-called 'old timer's disease'. Many famous people including Ronald Reagan, Charlton Heston and Iris Murdoch (as portrayed in the movie *Iris*) are openly mentioned as sufferers. Most of us know of someone with the disorder and frequently it is a family member. The personal and social costs are enormous.

Memory impairment in old age has long been recognised as common but until about 40 years ago it was usually regarded as a normal part of the ageing process – senescence. In the 1970s, post-mortem studies of the brains of older people who were senile when they died revealed that the microscopic appearances were those of Alzheimer's disease. Until this point, Alzheimer's disease was believed to be a rare condition afflicting people between 40 and 60 years of age. Named after the German neurologist, Alois Alzheimer, who first reported it in 1906, Alzheimer's disease was a footnote in medical textbooks.

There have been dramatic changes over the past 40 years. Alzheimer's disease and other dementias are now recognised as a major public health concern and have become the target of action plans at all levels of government. Although previously spurned by medical researchers, Alzheimer's disease is now the focus of numerous public and private research groups worldwide with attempts to identify causal factors, preventive measures, treatments and even cures. Textbooks, journals and conferences are now devoted entirely to Alzheimer's disease. Alzheimer's

Associations, organisations to support carers of people with dementia, have been formed worldwide.

In the past decade, drug treatments have become available, offering temporary improvement for some but hope for many. There is even anticipation of a vaccine. With this news, increasing numbers of people are presenting to their doctors with mild memory changes that in some cases represent the earliest symptoms of Alzheimer's disease. Interest in Alzheimer's disease is burgeoning.

Whether you know someone with Alzheimer's disease, are worried about your own memory, or just simply curious about the condition, this book is intended to meet your needs by providing an overview of Alzheimer's disease and other dementias. Case studies are used to illustrate the main points.

The book covers an array of topics. The early chapters set the scene by describing the various causes of memory impairment. In recent years much has been learnt about the risk factors for Alzheimer's disease and other dementias to the extent that plausible action can now be taken by most people during their early to mid-adult life that may reduce their risk of developing dementia in old age.

The common types of dementia are explained, particularly Alzheimer's disease, vascular dementia, frontotemporal dementia and dementia with Lewy bodies, and how they can be distinguished from each other. An important message is that there are many conditions that can affect memory that are potentially reversible, including stress, anxiety, depression and the effects of medication, alcohol and other drugs. Next the assessment process required to make an accurate diagnosis is outlined including the medical examination, memory tests, investigations and information required from collateral sources (usually family). While most medical centres would follow the same basic approach to assessment, there are quite significant individual differences that are mentioned. However, the crucial components are identified including the need to develop a collaborative management plan involving the person with dementia, family, doctors and other health care personnel.

The treatments available for dementia are covered in Chapters 7 and 8. With the advent of drug treatments for Alzheimer's disease and some other dementias, it is important to understand their indications and limitations. Some drugs are only designed to treat some of the psychological symptoms associated with dementia, for example, depression, anxiety and hallucinations. Others may improve memory and concentration.

The different types of drugs available are covered along with other naturopathic and herbal remedies. There are many psychosocial treatments used in dementia care; most are designed to improve the quality of life of the person with dementia and their carer. The fundamental approach is to adopt person-centred care. An overview of these therapies is provided including reality orientation, aromatherapy and music therapy to name a few.

As has been already implied, family caregivers are the linchpins around whom most dementia care is based. Without the support of family members and friends, it is difficult for the person with dementia to remain in their own home. Initially the support is largely emotional; in the later stages it is also physical. Caregiving can be both rewarding and stressful, often at the same time. Aspects of caregiving, including the important role of the Alzheimer's Association, are the focus of Chapter 9. Fortunately, formal community support provided by both government and non-government agencies has built considerably over the last 20 years. A plethora of services devoted to providing practical assistance around the home, respite for the caregiver, and activities for the person with dementia have been developed in order to allow home-based care to occur for as long as practicable. All services are based upon the principle of accurate assessment, both of the underlying cause of the mental decline and the actual needs of the person with dementia and their caregivers. Despite this, for most lay people the choice appears at times bewildering, at other times inadequate. Chapter 10 outlines the main types of services that are available in most developed countries.

For most persons with dementia, there comes a time when it is beyond the resources of family and formal community services to maintain them at home. There are various types of residential care options including hostels, special care units and nursing homes. Although often limited by availability, choosing the best option for the individual can be very difficult. Some hints are provided about how to make the choice. Staff of residential care face many of the same problems encountered by family caregivers – stress and frustration mixed with some job satisfaction. These and other residential care issues are covered in Chapter 11.

There are numerous ethical and legal considerations for a person with dementia, for example, power of attorney, ability to make a will, guardianship and ability to drive a car. In many situations, early planning with the involvement of the person with dementia can avoid snags later. When this hasn't been possible, the assessment of mental competency may

be required. While the actual legal process will vary between jurisdictions, the basic principles are the same. Ethical dilemmas are commonly encountered. What should we do when a person with dementia is living alone in squalid conditions and refuses all help? Should we tube feed people with severe dementia who are unable to swallow safely? These and other common problems are dealt with in Chapter 12.

In the final chapter I ponder the future of dementia care including the issues of prevention, early and pre-symptomatic diagnosis, and disease-altering therapies such as gene therapy, stem cell grafts and vaccines. I also consider the potential role of assistive technology in dementia care.

CHAPTER 1

What is Dementia?

We live in an ageing world. Over the last century global life expectancy at birth has increased from around 31 years in 1900 to 67.6 years in 2011, being higher in women (69.7 years) than men (65.6 years).[1] In developed countries life expectancy is even higher – 81.9 years in Australia, 81.5 years in Canada, 80.2 years in the UK, and 78.5 years in the US.[2] With more people living beyond their allotted 'three score years and ten', age-related conditions, including osteoarthritis, osteoporosis, cataracts, stroke, cancer, coronary artery disease and dementia, have increasingly impacted upon the health of our community. Of these conditions, dementia may be the condition that evokes the greatest fear in those contemplating the prospect of a lengthy old age. The possibility of becoming mentally incompetent, forgetful and dependent – in other words senile – can be very disturbing.

What is dementia?

First, let me clarify a few terms. 'Dementia' is a term used medically to describe a syndrome (set of symptoms) that is caused by many different diseases. These include Alzheimer's disease, vascular dementia, frontotemporal dementia, and dementia with Lewy bodies. An analogy is the term 'cancer' that is used to describe any malignant tumour but is not itself a specific disease. The answer to the frequently posed question, 'What is the difference between Alzheimer's disease and dementia?' is that, in a sense, there is no difference – Alzheimer's disease is one of the many different types of dementia.

The *dementia syndrome* is defined as an acquired decline in memory and thinking (cognition) due to brain disease that results in significant impairment of personal, social or occupational function. Other brain

13

functions that are affected include orientation, comprehension, calculating ability, learning capacity, language, judgement, reasoning and information processing. While there are some notable exceptions that I will discuss later, dementia is usually of gradual onset and progressive. The World Health Organization (WHO) *ICD-10* diagnostic criteria for dementia recommend that these symptoms and impairments be evident for at least six months before a confident diagnosis can be made.[3] While most dementias are currently irreversible, this does not mean that dementia is untreatable. The progression (course) can often be influenced and many symptoms can be ameliorated. As I discuss in later chapters, major advances have occurred over the last decade in this area.

Most dementias are progressive, and early symptoms and problems differ markedly from those in later stages. This may simply be a matter of degree – for example, mild memory impairment moving to profound memory impairment. Other symptoms and problems usually develop later in the course of the illness, urinary incontinence being one example. While it is customary to describe dementia in stages, there is overlap between stages and it may not always be easy to precisely state which stage a person has reached. The first stage is a 'pre-dementia' stage that has been named by some researchers as mild cognitive impairment. Currently we are unable to accurately and reliably identify what it constitutes but it basically means that the person is neither normal nor suffering from dementia but there is evidence of cognitive deterioration over time by either objective measurement (i.e. memory tests) and/or subjective decline reported by the person and/or informant. There is no impairment of basic activities of daily living (such as feeding, toileting, personal care) and minimal impairment of more complex higher-order functions (such as managing finances).[4] The next three stages, as commonly described to caregivers during a diagnostic assessment, are 'early' or 'mild', 'moderate' or 'middle', and 'late' or 'severe' dementia, respectively. The final stage, 'advanced dementia' is usually found only in nursing home residents. The stages, based on the course of Alzheimer's disease, should be regarded as a general guide as there is much variation (see Table 1.1).

Table 1.1 The stages of dementia

Stage	Clinical features
Pre-dementia, questionable dementia, or mild cognitive impairment	There is no set pattern and the various symptoms often occur independently of each other and are often only recognised retrospectively: • Subjective awareness of short-term memory deficits and/or close friends/relatives notice a mild change • Depression and anxiety along with other non-specific behaviour or memory changes • Personality changes such as apathy and irritability often attributed to age or depression • Close relationships might become strained, fewer social and hobby activities • Work performance, decision-making and problem-solving difficulties may occur
Mild or early dementia	Consistent deficits across a range of domains, however usually still able to function with minimal assistance: • Impairment in short-term memory interferes with day-to-day function, e.g. losing keys, forgetting conversations • Some disorientation in time, e.g. date, and may become disorientated when in unfamiliar places • Some word-finding difficulties – names, objects • Obvious difficulties with problem-solving, especially in novel situations • Difficulties in social functioning, for example, shopping, finances or business affairs, though may superficially appear normal and engage in them • More difficult household tasks no longer done and less interest in hobbies • May require prompting in personal care

cont.

Stage	Clinical features
Moderate or middle-stage dementia	More severe deficits, clearly needs assistance from a caregiver to function at a level comparable to before onset of dementia: • Severe memory loss and rapidly forgets new information • Usually disoriented in time and often place • Obvious difficulties in finding words, often doesn't speak spontaneously • Starts to misidentify familiar people • Problem-solving and judgement very poor • Unable to function independently in social situations, but is usually able to attend with supervision • Only able to perform simple chores at home • Requires assistance with personal care • Behavioural difficulties emerge, for example, wandering, agitation, aggression, psychosis, sleep disturbance
Severe or late-stage dementia	No semblance of independent function so the majority of persons with severe dementia are in residential care: • Very severe memory loss, only fragments remain • Oriented to person (i.e. they know who they are but not the place or the time) • Unable to solve problems or make judgements • Language skills limited to a few words and phrases • Regularly misidentifies familiar people • Social function is minimal even with supervision • No significant self-care capacity • Frequent incontinence • Behavioural difficulties increase

Stage	Clinical features
Advanced dementia	Completely dependent on caregivers for all aspects of daily living • No semblance of memory function • Usually inarticulate, may be mute • Cannot identify familiar people • Very poor comprehension of simple verbal commands • Social interactions virtually non-existent • May lose capacity to stand, walk and sit up • Incontinent of urine and faeces

How does dementia differ from normal ageing?

Unlike dementia, the concept of normal ageing is poorly understood. Many of the accompaniments of ageing that result in disabilities such as cancer, prostate disease and hormonal deficiencies have become treatable, which challenges the notion that they are inevitable features of the physiological ageing process and suggests that they may be considered pathologic conditions. Efforts to characterise mental changes intrinsic to normal ageing are fraught with difficulty, with terms such as 'benign senescent forgetfulness', 'age-associated memory impairment', and 'age-associated cognitive decline' being used now to generally reflect the extremes of normal ageing rather than describing a precursor of pathologic ageing.

We acquire knowledge through an active cognitive processing of information that involves thinking, learning and remembering; it is known as 'fluid intelligence'. Fluid intelligence tends to decline with age. Short-term memory wanes to a degree, but in contrast to a person with dementia who will tend to forget the whole experience, the normal older person will only forget parts of the experience. For example, where the person with dementia might forget altogether having been to the cinema, the normal older person might just forget some details of the film. New learning becomes more difficult for the normal older person, the ability to solve novel problems declines and the speed of mental processing slows. There is a speed–accuracy trade off, however, with the older person tending to make fewer errors.[5]

There is also an age-related tendency to have some increased difficulty in word-finding and remembering names – a situation that most of us have experienced as having a word 'on the tip of the tongue'. In most cases, the missing word appears a bit later without prompting. Associated anxiety about not getting the word out may often magnify the problem. In addition, those people who are more 'tongue-tied' than others and have always had some difficulties in expressing themselves find that the ageing process exacerbates this tendency.

The accumulation as one ages of all the knowledge and products of previous cognitive processes is known as 'crystallised intelligence'. Crystallised intelligence does not decline in normal ageing; rather, it often increases with maturity and brings greater wisdom. It is one of the reasons that societal elders are held in high regard and hold senior positions in most cultures.[6]

There is no precise point at which these normal age-related cognitive changes become a pathological entity (disease). And there is considerable debate on the issue in the scientific community, particularly regarding those aged 90 years and over where research has been very limited. There are, however, some warning signs. Normal age-related decline takes place over decades, so decline over a shorter time – months or a few years – is liable to be pathological. This is particularly the case if the person's functional performance has declined relative to their peers and they are unable to adapt to maintain functioning in normal life.

What are the main types of dementia?

Alzheimer's disease is the most common type of dementia and accounts for about 50 to 75 per cent of dementia cases, sometimes occurring in combination with other dementias. Vascular dementia is the next most common accounting for 20 to 30 per cent of cases although it is probably more common in South East and East Asian countries. Mixed Alzheimer's–vascular dementia is probably more widespread than clinical diagnoses would suggest with some post-mortem studies suggesting that it might involve as much as 25 per cent of dementia cases. Frontotemporal dementia, which includes Pick's disease, occurs in approximately 5 to 10 per cent of cases and is particularly common in younger age groups. Over the past 15 years, dementia with Lewy bodies has become increasingly recognised and is said to account for up to 5 per cent of cases, though it is possible that up to another 15 per cent may have it in combination with Alzheimer's disease.[7]

Numerous other conditions can cause dementia, but most of them are rare. Conditions such as alcohol abuse, hypothyroidism, vitamin B_{12} deficiency and Parkinson's disease are regularly found in persons with dementia but in most cases the main cause of the dementia is Alzheimer's disease or vascular dementia. Well-known less common causes of dementia include brain tumours, normal pressure hydrocephalus, progressive supranuclear palsy, cerebral vasculitis and brain trauma. In younger age groups, human immunodeficiency virus (HIV)-related disorders are a more prominent cause, though it should be stressed that in most cases, other HIV-related disorders have been previously diagnosed and the dementia occurs late in the course of the disease.

How common is dementia?

To date, over 100 studies worldwide have reported on the prevalence of dementia. Prevalence is the proportion of people in a population that has the disease at a defined time point or period. Dementia is an age-related condition and under the age of 60 it is quite rare occurring in around 0.1 per cent of the population, but because the baby boomer bulge is currently in this age-bracket, the number of new dementia cases with symptoms commencing before age 65 has increased considerably in recent years. The prevalence of dementia doubles every five years from the age of 60, with less than 2 per cent of 60 to 64-year-olds and over 20 per cent of those aged 85 years and over having dementia. According to the World Alzheimer Report, the global prevalence of dementia in 2011 was 36 million people.[8] Incidence refers to the rate at which new cases occur in a population and this also increases with age. Worldwide it is uncertain how many new cases of dementia occur each year, but in Australia in 2009 it was estimated that there were 69,600 new cases per year,[9] while in 2005 in England and Wales it was estimated that there were 180,000 new cases per year.[10]

Is dementia becoming more common?

The simple answer to this question is 'yes', but the increase is basically due to the ageing of the population, not to any innate changes in the risk of developing dementia. As more people survive or avoid early and midlife illnesses such as cardiac and infectious diseases, they live to an age where they are at higher risk of dementia. This is accentuated by the survival of increasing numbers of persons aged over 85 years – the age group at greatest risk.

Until recently there was no evidence to suggest that there had been any significant change in the risk of developing dementia at any particular age. However in 2012, a major epidemiological study of dementia from Rotterdam in the Netherlands reported that there had been a non-significant reduction of dementia incidence between 1990 and 2005 although the reasons for this were unclear.[11] What is not known is whether there have been any changes compared with a hundred or more years ago, or whether the incidence will change in 20 years or more. The impact on rates of dementia of altering various lifestyle risk factors, as described in Chapters 2 and 3, is also unknown. Yet, computer modelling we have undertaken in our research group, under the leadership of Dr Victor Vickland, has demonstrated that if it were possible to delay the onset of dementia by two years by a hypothetical intervention introduced in Australia in 2020, the prevalence of dementia would be reduced by 13 per cent by 2050, while a five-year delay of dementia onset would reduce the prevalence by 30 per cent by 2050.[12]

One factor that may impact upon the prevalence of dementia is the introduction about 15 years ago of cholinesterase inhibitor drugs such as donepezil (Aricept), galantamine (Reminyl) or rivastigmine (Exelon) that are now being prescribed for Alzheimer's disease (see Chapter 7). These agents appear to slow the progress of the disease for around 12–18 months in approximately 50 to 60 per cent of patients. Their long-term effects are unclear and while it is most likely that they do not alter the course of the disease, there is some limited evidence that they might slow disease progression.[13] If the course of Alzheimer's disease is prolonged, the prevalence of dementia will increase simply because more people are surviving with the illness. Thus the duration of Alzheimer's disease being increased by one year would have a similar but opposite effect to delaying its onset. In other words, the prevalence of dementia cases might increase by some tens of thousands! It will be some years before it is known whether these agents have any measurable impact upon disease duration.

The Australian Institute of Health and Welfare estimated that 298,000 Australians had dementia in 2011 of whom 70 per cent lived in the community. Based on projections of population ageing and growth, there will be almost 900,000 people with dementia in Australia by 2050, about a threefold increase. This marked increase in dementia cases is mainly attributable to the projected increase in the number of persons surviving to age 80 and beyond.[14]

These projections are not unique to Australia. Other developed migrant countries such as Canada, USA and New Zealand will see a similar pattern. North America, with an estimated 4.38 million people with dementia in 2010, will have around a 150 per cent increase in dementia prevalence to have approximately 11 million people with dementia in 2050. Western European countries, such as the UK, with stable populations, will have less dramatic changes although the prevalence of dementia will still increase by about 93 per cent from 2010 to 2050, increasing from around 9.95 million to 18.65 million people. It is in the developing world where the most dramatic increases will occur between 2010 and 2050 with 311 per cent growth in east Asia, 304 per cent in south Asia, 435 per cent in central Latin America, and 438 per cent in North Africa and the Middle East.[15]

What is the impact of dementia upon society?

The global impact of dementia is growing. According to the WHO Global Burden of Disease Report updated to 2004, dementia was ranked as the second leading cause of years lived with a disability for those aged 60 years and over (blindness is number one) and the eighth cause of years of life lost (heart disease, cancer and stroke are the top three).[16] In developed countries, cognitive impairment is by far the strongest health condition predictor of institutionalisation. In low and middle-income countries, research from the 10/66 Dementia Research Group in Cuba, Dominican Republic, Venezuela, Peru, China, India and Mexico has found that dementia is the leading cause of both disability and dependency followed by limb weakness, stroke, depression, eyesight problems and arthritis.[17]

According to the World Alzheimer Report 2010, the costs associated with dementia totalled US$604 billion, about 1 per cent of global GDP, but in high-income countries this represented 1.24 per cent of GDP.[18] If dementia care were a company, it would be the largest in the world. These costs can be divided into three components: the direct costs of medical care, the direct costs of social care (such as community care packages and residential care), and the costs of informal care (unpaid care provided by families and others). The World Alzheimer Report 2010 estimated that 42 per cent of costs were accounted for by informal care, another 42 per cent by social care, and 16 per cent by medical care. It also tentatively estimated an 85 per cent increase in costs to 2030 just based on the increase in numbers of people with dementia.[19] In Australia, Access Economics

released a report for Alzheimer's Australia in 2009 which estimated that dementia will become the third greatest source of health and aged care expenditure in Australia within about two decades, and that by the 2060s, dementia will far exceed expenditure on any other health condition.[20] Similarly a 2010 report commissioned by the Alzheimer's Research Trust in the UK estimated that the annual societal cost of dementia (£23 billion) almost matched those of cancer (£12 billion), heart disease (£8 billion) and stroke (£5 billion) combined.[21] In the US, it was estimated that the total monetary cost of dementia in 2010 was between $157 billion and $215 billion, of which Medicare paid about $11 billion.[22]

Dementia already has a considerable effect upon the community. The projected massive increase in the number of dementia cases over the next 40 years is likely to further elevate dementia in the list of leading causes of disease burden, though current and future therapies may ameliorate the impact. The Global Burden of Disease 2010 study released in December 2012 reported that in 2010 dementia was now the 11th leading cause of Disability Adjusted Life Years lost in Western Europe and the 12th in high income North America across all age groups, much higher than it had been in earlier reports.[23] Such a striking increase, with the need for more medical, community and residential services, will have huge economic consequences just to maintain current standards. The dilemma of how to fund such demands from the public purse has been a concern of economists, health care planners and politicians for some time. The move towards self-funded retirement and user-pays principles in provision of services has largely evolved from this.

In Australia, these concerns led to dementia becoming a National Health Priority in 2006 with an associated national strategy. Other countries such as the UK, France, Denmark, Norway, South Korea and the US have subsequently announced national strategies. The National Dementia Strategy in the UK was released in 2009 and involves a five-year plan built around three key steps: ensuring better knowledge of dementia and removing stigma; ensuring early diagnosis, support and treatment for people with dementia and their family and carers; and developing services to meet changing needs better.[24] The strategy was well received although the Alzheimer's Society and the Alzheimer's Research Trust issued a public statement later in the year calling for a tripling of the UK's annual investment in dementia research by 2014.[25]

In the US, President Obama signed the National Alzheimer's Project Act in January 2011 that was designed to coordinate clinical care, residential

and home care and research as part of a national plan to cope with the dementia epidemic. Subsequently in February 2012 additional funding was announced for research, training, and public education. In May 2012 the director of the National Institutes of Health announced a research programme that aimed to stop and reverse Alzheimer's disease by 2025.[26]

Summary

The dementia syndrome is an acquired decline in memory and thinking due to brain disease that results in significant impairment of personal, social or occupational function. It is not due to a normal ageing process. The most common type of dementia is Alzheimer's disease, though other common types include vascular dementia, frontotemporal dementia and dementia with Lewy bodies. Dementia is increasing in prevalence due to the ageing population and is projected to have a commensurate increase in its economic impact and burden of disease in our society. In recognition of the increasing impact of dementia upon society, many countries have announced national dementia strategies in recent years.

Prevention of Dementia

General Strategies

'How can I stop myself from getting dementia?' is a question commonly posed to dementia specialists. Until recently, it has not been possible to provide any advice based on reputable research. The situation is rapidly changing, however, and in this and the next chapter I describe the known risk factors for dementia and strategies that may counteract them. But it is also sobering to note that in April 2010, the National Institutes of Health in the US held a 'State of the Science' conference on preventing Alzheimer's disease and cognitive decline, issuing a statement that there was no evidence of even moderate scientific quality supporting the association of any modifiable factor with reduced risk of Alzheimer's disease.[1] This is largely due to the methodological challenges inherent in gathering high-quality evidence for prevention of illnesses that take many years to develop and are likely to have multiple factors contributing to the aetiology.[2] So, while there are strong hints in the research about what might help, no strategy is proven to work.

One of the features of recent research has been the convergence of identified risk factors for the two most common types of dementia – Alzheimer's disease and vascular dementia. Thus, I discuss prevention strategies for dementia as a whole and will indicate where particular strategies may be important for specific types of dementia.

Disease prevention

It is important to appreciate that intentional efforts to prevent any disease imply that there is some reasonable understanding of what causes it. The disease process by which the causal factors turn a normal state into a pathological (diseased) state must also be understood. Recognition of 'risk

factors' that may facilitate or are associated with the disease process, and 'protective factors' that may suppress the process or are associated with normality is also crucial. Risk and protective factors may include genetic, medical, biological, environmental, dietary, social and cultural aspects. In the field of dementia, it has only been over the last decade that knowledge has grown sufficiently in these domains for prevention strategies to be mounted.

Historically, of course, many conditions have been prevented unintentionally or by unknown methods. An example is suicide in Australian men aged between 45 and 75 years where annual rates have been steadily declining since the mid 1960s.[3] No specific suicide prevention strategies were responsible for the change. While it has been hypothesised that the change may be related to improvements in the general health of men in this age group, no one knows for sure what has been responsible, particularly as suicide rates in younger men have increased dramatically during the same period and those in men aged over 75 years remain very high.

Disease prevention may involve either elimination or postponement of the disease.

Disease elimination

Disease elimination suits diseases with single known causes (pathogens) that can be specifically targeted in a prevention strategy. This has been the model used in infectious diseases such as smallpox, which was eliminated from the community by population vaccination programmes, and in other diseases such as measles, rubella, polio and diphtheria, which can be prevented in most individuals by vaccinations. This will also be the model used in proposed gene therapies for genetic disorders where there is a single gene mutation responsible for the disease. The gene therapy will target the mutation and correct the abnormality before it has had sufficient opportunity to cause irreparable damage. Another method of disease elimination involves DNA testing of a foetus during early pregnancy where a known genetic risk for a disorder exists allowing for the option of a termination of the pregnancy.

As most cases of dementia are likely to be multifactorial in origin, disease elimination is not a realistic objective of prevention strategies unless the strategy targets a 'final common pathway' of the disease process. Hopes were raised in 1999 by the publication in the prestigious journal *Nature* of reports of immunotherapy treatment that eliminated beta-amyloid plaques, the major pathological abnormality in the brain in Alzheimer's

disease (see Chapter 5). The therapy stimulated the immune system of mice to identify and assault the amyloid plaques.[4] As Alzheimer's disease does not naturally occur in mice, the research involved the transplantation of a rare human Alzheimer's disease gene into the mouse. Immunisation of young transplanted mice with a protein named AN-1792 prevented the development of the beta-amyloid plaques, while immunisation of older mice after they had already developed beta-amyloid plaques resulted in stopping the further accumulation of beta-amyloid protein and in some cases reversed the process. Later independent studies showed that AN-1792 also improved the performance of these mice on tests designed to measure rodent memory. Once these results hit the media, AN-1792 was quickly dubbed the Alzheimer 'vaccine' (although this is an inaccurate description, with immunotherapy being a better term).

These exciting findings quickly led to human trials of AN-1792 with the approval of both the US Food and Drug Administration (FDA) and the UK Medicines Control Agency. Initial trials in 2000 to test its safety in humans (known as Phase I trials) revealed no problems and led to the commencement in 2001 of a small Phase IIA trial in Europe and the US to begin assessing the drug's effectiveness, to determine the best dosage, and to further test safety. The trial enrolled 360 people with mild to moderate Alzheimer's disease. In January 2002, the sponsors, Elan and Wyeth-Ayerst Laboratories, announced suspension of the dosing schedule after four participants who had received multiple doses of AN-1792 developed symptoms of inflammation of the central nervous system. By the end of February 2002, the number of affected participants had increased to 15 with several deaths and the trial was discontinued in March 2002.[5]

Even if these concerns about the safety of AN-1792 are resolved, there are other concerns. A hypothetical safety concern is the possibility that by provoking an immune reaction to one of the body's own proteins, AN-1792 could stimulate an autoimmune reaction in which the body mobilises an indiscriminate onslaught on its own tissues. Also, more recent studies in mice have found an increased risk of cerebral haemorrhage (stroke) in vaccinated mice. A follow-up study was conducted 4.6 years after immunisation involving 129 participants that were immunised and 30 that were on placebo. Approximately 20 per cent of the participants that were immunised were classified as antibody responders and these participants were found to have had significantly less functional decline than placebo-treated participants. No further cases of encephalitis were recorded.[6]

In June 2012, researchers from the Karolinska Institute in Sweden announced in the journal *Lancet Neurology* that a new active vaccine CAD106 had positive effects. They found that over the three years of the study, 80 per cent of the patients involved in the trials developed their own protective antibodies against beta-amyloid without suffering any side effects. Now larger studies will be mounted to test the efficacy of the vaccine.[7] So, while there are tantalising suggestions that immunotherapy might provide a therapeutic opportunity to eliminate Alzheimer's disease, it is clearly not going to happen just yet. I explore this theme further in Chapter 13.

Disease postponement

In complex or chronic diseases associated with ageing such as dementia, disease postponement may be an adequate prevention measure for the foreseeable future. While postponement only delays the onset of the disease, the period of time involved can still have a dramatic effect. Delaying the onset of dementia could allow a person to enjoy a longer period of healthy life, before succumbing to some other condition perhaps before dementia developed or when their dementia is still relatively mild. The computer modelling by our team led by Victor Vickland indicates that if we were able to delay the onset of dementia by five years commencing in 2010, by 2040 there would be over 260,000 fewer cases of dementia in Australia than would occur without such delay.[8] A secure web-based application based at Johns Hopkins University in Baltimore allows similar calculations to be made for the US and other countries (available at: www. biostat.jhsph.edu/project/globalAD). Using the state of Maryland as an example, the effect of preventative interventions that could delay the onset of Alzheimer's disease by two years from 2015 is to decrease the prevalence of Alzheimer's disease in 2030 by approximately 22 per cent.[9]

Disease postponement is largely about modifying known risk factors of dementia. In 2011, researchers Deborah Barnes and Kristine Yaffe from San Francisco published in *Lancet Neurology* the potential benefit of targeting seven potentially modifiable risk factors for Alzheimer's disease: diabetes, midlife hypertension, midlife obesity, smoking, depression, cognitive inactivity or low educational attainment, and physical inactivity. They estimated that up to a half of Alzheimer's disease cases worldwide (approximately 17.2 million) were potentially attributable to these factors and that a 10–25 per cent reduction in all seven risk factors could potentially prevent as many as 1.1–3.0 million Alzheimer's disease cases

worldwide.[10] I will address prevention by reviewing these and other risk factors.

Public health model of prevention

The public health model of prevention identifies three types of strategy to prevent disease. *Universal strategies* apply to the whole population, *selective strategies* to individuals at high risk, and *indicated strategies* to individuals with early symptoms or indications of disease. These different types of strategy can be applied to dementia prevention. The rest of this chapter outlines some universal strategies; the next chapter covers selective and indicated strategies of dementia prevention.

Universal dementia prevention strategies

Universal strategies for disease prevention are applied to everybody in a population because all of the population is at potential risk of harm from the targeted risk factor. Common examples include water purification to eliminate waterborne infectious diseases in the water supply, hand washing before food handling to prevent bacterial food contamination, and treatment of sewage before disposal to prevent bacterial contamination of waterways. Although universal strategies may seem to have only a limited effect for the individual, when applied across a whole population the effect is magnified considerably. A number of dementia risk factors apply to the whole population, so universal strategies are applicable.

Early childhood environment

It is often said that the early years of life are the most important for human development. There is now mounting evidence that childhood experiences may influence the risk of an individual developing dementia.[11, 12] Adverse childhood events include sexual abuse, physical abuse, emotional abuse, parental death, malnourishment, hardship and illness. These may impact upon brain development and there is evidence of structural brain changes in young and middle-aged individuals who have experienced adverse childhood events.[13] Furthermore, in childhood there is strong evidence of associated cognitive dysfunction, with some studies showing persistence into adulthood.[14] This could impact upon brain reserve in late life as described later in this chapter.

Several studies have demonstrated that there is an increased risk of dementia associated with a history of early parental death even when

other factors are taken into account.[15] However, the relationship between aspects of the childhood environment and dementia is variable and likely to interact with genetic and other factors. Positive experiences might be protective, while some who have been the victims of abuses and hardship are resilient, coping through friendships, sport, education and work. Indeed, this provides some indirect support for some of the strategies described later in this chapter that might reduce dementia risk. This is a field of research attracting more attention, although the difficulties in obtaining accurate childhood information not contaminated by faulty recall of older participants has hindered progress.

Age and the role of antioxidants and nutrition

Increasing age is the most well-established risk factor for dementia and the risk continues to increase after the age of 90.[16] It remains unclear whether the increased rates of dementia in old age are caused by the ageing process itself or because of other diseases or events that are themselves age-related. Obviously we do not want to prevent a person from getting older, but a better understanding of the ageing process and of factors that enhance its effects may lead to some useful prevention strategies.

One particular strategy involving the ingestion of antioxidants may already be informally in place. Antioxidants potentially have a role in preventing dementia. As the brain ages, its capacity to remove certain small molecules known as 'free radicals' is reduced, resulting in cell death and increased susceptibility of nerve cells to other factors that cause damage, including inflammation. The brain cells' natural defences against this damage include manufacturing antioxidants that mop up free radicals, but with age some of these protective mechanisms decline.

Curcumin (from the herb turmeric), alpha-lipoic acid, flavonoids, vitamin B_6, vitamin C, vitamin E and vitamin A are just a few of the many antioxidants available on the shelves in health food stores. A number of these have been examined for their ability to prevent Alzheimer's disease, vascular dementia, or cognitive impairment, but the results so far are equivocal.

Vitamins C and E

There is modest and inconsistent evidence that vitamins C and E may have a protective role. The Honolulu-Asia Ageing Study found that older men who took supplements of vitamins C and E had lower rates of vascular

dementia and cognitive impairment but not Alzheimer's disease.[17] An epidemiological study published in the influential *Journal of the American Medical Association (JAMA)* in June 2002 suggested that eating foods rich in antioxidants (such as fibres, grains, fish, green vegetables) especially vitamin E (but not vitamin E supplements) may help lower the risk of developing Alzheimer's disease.[18] Another study published in the *Archives of Neurology* in July 2002 found vitamin E to be protective against memory decline.[19]

The optimal dose of vitamin E is not known. Many doctors recommend 400 International Units twice daily because it is safe for most individuals and it should have the antioxidant effect desired in the brain, although there have been concerns about increased mortality on higher doses. People taking anticoagulants like warfarin may not be able to take vitamin E or will need to be monitored closely by their doctor.

A review of the prevention of dementia published in the *Archives of Neurology* in October 2009 concluded that the research on the effects of vitamin E and vitamin C was unclear, particularly as evidence from randomised controlled trials has been inconsistent with most studies finding no relationship between vitamin E supplementation and cognitive performance.[20] Recent studies continue to demonstrate inconsistent results with a Dutch study showing benefit from vitamin E but not vitamin C and a German study having the opposite findings with benefit from vitamin C but not vitamin E.[21, 22] There is currently insufficient evidence to support the view that vitamin E or C supplements will prevent Alzheimer's disease.

Curcumin

Curcumin is a polyphenol compound derived from turmeric, used a lot in Indian cuisine, that has diverse biological properties that include binding to beta-amyloid plaques to inhibit amyloid accumulation and aggregation, and inhibition of alpha synuclein aggregation in Parkinson's disease.[23] A recently published 24-week randomised, double-blind, placebo-controlled study of oral curcumin showed no clinical effect in subjects with mild to moderate Alzheimer's disease. Curcumin was well tolerated but there was a suggestion that it did not reach adequate bioavailability.[24] Of course this was a treatment rather than a prevention trial so more work is needed to see whether curcumin has a role in preventing Alzheimer's disease and other degenerative disorders.

Alcohol (red wine)

It has been well established that excessive alcohol intake, usually in combination with thiamine deficiency, can cause brain damage. One well-known type of brain damage is the Wernicke-Korsakoff syndrome due to thiamine deficiency in which profound short-term memory impairment occurs. This is not a progressive condition, providing alcohol consumption ceases and the thiamine is replaced, but it still leaves the sufferer severely impaired. Alcohol-related dementia is more controversial as precise brain pathology has not been established but alcohol does appear to be neurotoxic in excess amounts. The possible risk appears to be mainly in persons under the age of 60 years.[25] A recent study of younger-onset dementia (onset before age 65) we conducted in eastern Sydney found that alcohol was a contributing factor to around 20 per cent of cases, with the average age of onset of symptoms in the early 50s.[26]

Epidemiological studies have not demonstrated that alcohol is a risk factor for dementia in older people. Indeed, as demonstrated in the Rotterdam Study, light-to-moderate drinking (one to three drinks per day) was significantly associated with a *lower* risk of any dementia, and vascular dementia in particular, in individuals aged 55 years or older.[27] The effect seemed to be unchanged by the source of alcohol. However, some studies have suggested that red wine may have particular benefit. The flavonoids in wine – powerful antioxidant substances also contained in tea, fruits and vegetables – have been thought to offer protection. One study has found that the intake of antioxidant flavonoids was inversely related to the risk of dementia,[28] and a second has reported in an eight-week double-blind randomised control trial that consumption of high cocoa flavanols improved cognition in older people with mild cognitive impairment (MCI).[29] The benefits of alcohol might also be restricted to individuals who do not have the Alzheimer's disease associated apolipoprotein E ε4 allele (form) of the gene (see Chapter 3).[30]

While these findings may give some encouragement to drink alcohol in old age, a few words of caution are required. For some individuals there may be a fine line between a potentially beneficial amount of alcohol and a deleterious amount. Further, women experience the deleterious effects of alcohol at much lower amounts than men. This uncertainty was emphasised in two reports from the 2012 Alzheimer's Association International Conference in Vancouver. Researchers from San Francisco presented a 20-year study of 1300 women aged 65 and older and reported that moderate alcohol consumption in women was not protective against dementia.

Furthermore, women who increased their alcohol consumption over the course of the study had an increased risk of developing dementia.[31] The second study found that men and women aged 65 years from the US who were binge drinking at least once per month had an increased risk of cognitive decline over an eight-year period.[32]

Until prospective controlled studies of light-to-moderate alcohol intake are undertaken, it remains an unproven preventive strategy. In those who have established dementia, relatively small amounts of alcohol can cause increased confusion and behavioural changes.

Vitamin B$_{12}$, vitamin B$_6$ and folate – the role of homocysteine

Vitamin B$_{12}$ (cobalamin), vitamin B$_6$ (pyridoxine) and folate play vital roles in effective DNA synthesis and normal brain metabolism. These B group vitamins act as catalysts in chemical reactions in which homocysteine is converted to methionine, and dietary deficiencies can result in a build-up of serum homocysteine. High levels of homocysteine have been linked with Alzheimer's disease, vascular dementia, cerebrovascular disease and cognitive impairment in general. In addition, deficiencies in vitamin B$_{12}$, vitamin B$_6$ and folate are known to cause depression and other neurological syndromes.[33] What is unclear at present is whether these associations reflect a causal mechanism between homocysteine and dementia. However recent research from Oxford University has provided some better evidence of a link. In a two-year randomised placebo-controlled trial of administering daily vitamin B$_{12}$, vitamin B$_6$ and folate tablets to patients with mild cognitive impairment, the B vitamins were found to halve the rate of brain shrinkage as shown on the patients' brain scans and it was found that that the patients who had the least shrinkage did better on memory tests.[34]

There is also some evidence that homocysteine may exacerbate cognitive impairment after acute stroke, so there may be an additive effect. Certainly, homocysteine provides another link between Alzheimer's disease and cerebrovascular disease, but the extent to which it may be responsible for either condition is not known.

Probably the most important issue is that there is a simple treatment for preventing high levels of homocysteine. A diet rich in green leafy vegetables, low fat dairy products, citrus fruits and juices, wholewheat bread, and dry beans can significantly lower levels of homocysteine. Since 1998 in the US, the FDA has required the addition of folate to enriched breads, cereals, flours, corn meals, pastas, rice and other grain products but it is too soon to know whether this will reduce the rate of dementia.

In countries like Australia where folate enhancement of grain products does not routinely occur, folate supplements could also be considered. In individuals with normal folate levels but elevated homocysteine levels, low-dose B-group vitamin supplementation that includes vitamin B_{12}, vitamin B_6 and folate (50 micrograms daily) should suffice, while individuals with folate deficiency may require up to 5 milligrams daily until the deficiency is overcome before reverting to a lower dose. Of course, specific vitamin B_{12} replacement is required if that vitamin is deficient.

It is unlikely that these vitamins are harmful (apart from concerns that folate enhancement in pregnant women might be associated with an increased risk of asthma in their children)[35] and may have other cardiovascular benefits anyway.

Fish – omega-3 polyunsaturated fatty acids

Oily fish, such as salmon, mackerel, herring and sardines are a rich source of omega-3 polyunsaturated fatty acids (PUFA) which are essential for brain development and have a protective effect against cardiovascular disease and therefore the vascular risk factors implied in vascular dementia and in Alzheimer's disease. There is also evidence that omega-3 PUFA can be neuroprotective and may have a role in neurotransmission.[36] Observational studies have suggested beneficial effects of fish consumption. A French study reported that the consumption of fish at least once per week reduces the risk of dementia by one third over a seven-year period. Education may have been a confounding factor as more highly educated older people were eating more fish.[37] A recent Cochrane Collaboration review of three randomised trials of omega-3 PUFA supplementation in cognitively healthy older adults found no benefit on cognitive function in the trials that ranged from 6 to 40 months duration. The reviewers concluded that longer studies were required. The main reported adverse effects were mild gastrointestinal symptoms. So, at present there is no convincing evidence that omega-3 PUFA prevent dementia but there may be other health benefits.[38]

The 'Mediterranean diet'

The 'Mediterranean diet' (see Table 2.1) is not actually a diet but essentially a dietary pattern based on those found in Greece, Crete and southern Italy in the 1960s where life expectancy was high and cardiovascular diseases low. It brings together many of the previously mentioned dietary components involving a high intake of plant foods including nuts, fruits,

cereals and legumes, fresh vegetables full of antioxidants, fish, olive oil (or other monounsaturated fats), and low to moderate amounts of red wine. The dietary pattern avoids saturated and trans fats, has little red meat, and encourages physical activity. In many respects, the Mediterranean diet is similar to the food guide pyramid popularised in the US in the 1990s. Fortunately, it is a dietary pattern that is very palatable.[39, 40]

Table 2.1 The Mediterranean diet

High consumption (daily)

Grains/Carbohydrates: breads, pasta, rice, potatoes, couscous, polenta
Fruits: 2–4 servings
Vegetables: 3–5 servings of different varieties including dark green leafy vegetables
Legumes, nuts (almonds, walnuts), beans, garlic, onions, herbs
Dairy Products: mainly yoghurt (low fat preferred), cheese (low fat and feta preferred), small amounts of low fat or skimmed milk

Moderate consumption (a few times per week)

Fish (grilled or steamed)
Poultry
Eggs: maximum 4 per week
Extra virgin olive oil (canola or peanut oil can substitute) – on salad, vegetables
Red wine: 1–2 standard drinks for women, 2–3 standard drinks for men with meals (purple grape juice is an alternative for teetotallers)

Low consumption (a few times per month)

Red meat – lean with no visible fat
Sweets

Avoid

Foods high in saturated fats and trans fats (e.g. snack foods, processed peanut butter)
Processed foods
Butter
Margarine
Lard

There is evidence that this dietary pattern is associated with better cognition in late life but there are some contradictory findings. A prospective study from New York published in the *Journal of the American Medical Association* in 2009 found that high adherence to the Mediterranean diet was associated with a lower risk of developing Alzheimer's disease.[41] In contrast, a study from Bordeaux, France published in the same issue of the journal reported that while high adherence to the Mediterranean diet slowed cognitive decline, it was not associated with a reduced risk of developing dementia.[42] The type of fats in the Mediterranean dietary pattern may be a critical component. A recent study that followed up over 6000 older women over four years found that higher saturated fat intake was associated with worse global cognitive trajectories, whereas higher monounsaturated fat intake was related to better trajectories.[43] There is also evidence that the Mediterranean dietary pattern is associated with increased longevity and a lower risk of developing the metabolic syndrome, a condition that has also been identified as a risk factor for dementia (see Chapter 3).[44, 45]

The evidence for the effectiveness of antioxidants and nutritional factors in the prevention of dementia is improving but is difficult to obtain in a definitive way. This is due to the challenges in running the types of large studies required involving thousands of subjects monitored over many years to determine whether particular antioxidants or dietary patterns may be effective. There is sufficient evidence, however, to guide us towards a dietary pattern that has overall health benefits even if it is unclear whether it might prevent dementia.

Vitamin D

Vitamin D might reduce the risk of dementia indirectly by lowering the risk of diseases that often precede dementia such as cardiovascular disease and cerebrovascular disease. In addition it might have a role in clearing beta-amyloid plaques, in reducing inflammation in the brain and in stimulating nerve regeneration. Most vitamin D is made by the body through the skin's exposure to sunlight and it can also be found in foods such as oily fish. Vitamin D is vital for bone strength as it assists in the absorption of calcium. High rates of vitamin D deficiency in older adults have been reported in studies from Europe and the US.[46]

A recent systematic review of studies examining the association between cognitive impairment and vitamin D deficiency found that while there was an increased risk of cognitive impairment in individuals with low vitamin D levels, the quality of the studies was poor with too many

confounding issues. The authors felt that there was insufficient evidence to warrant vitamin D supplementation on the current evidence and that there needed to be placebo-controlled randomised trials showing benefit before supplementation could be recommended.[47]

Caffeine

Whether or not this is the best section to deal with caffeine is debatable – while for some of us caffeine is a major nutrient, there may be argument about it! There has long been evidence in the test tube that caffeine may have a potential role in treating Alzheimer's disease. Caffeine belongs to a family of chemicals that include drugs such as propentofylline, a drug that has been investigated as a treatment for Alzheimer's disease. Propentofylline acts by modulating the activity of glial cells in the brain. Caffeine itself has also been shown to stimulate nerve cells to take in more choline, the building block for acetylcholine, which is the most important neurotransmitter for memory function. Caffeine also blocks receptors for adenosine, another neurotransmitter, a function thought to be of potential therapeutic benefit in Alzheimer's disease. There is also evidence that in transgenic mice, caffeine reduces levels of brain beta-amyloid protein.[48]

The clinical evidence that caffeine consumption might be associated with lower rates of Alzheimer's disease is limited to a case-control study. The study has numerous weaknesses but does point to the need for larger, prospective studies.[49] At this stage, however, there is insufficient evidence to recommend the use of caffeine to prevent Alzheimer's disease. It should be remembered that caffeine can have adverse effects on sleep and on the heart and can increase anxiety.

Education, intelligence and brain reserve

Low levels of formal education have been found to be associated with higher levels of cognitive impairment, dementia in general and Alzheimer's disease in particular. Another way of looking at it is that people with higher levels of education are less likely to develop dementia, approximately halving the risk.[50] Worldwide, low education has been estimated to be responsible for 19 per cent of Alzheimer's disease cases and it is estimated that a 10 per cent reduction in prevalence of low education worldwide could potentially reduce the number of cases of Alzheimer's disease by 534,000.[51]

The mechanism of this relationship between education and dementia is unclear but there are a number of possibilities. One possibility is that a low level of education may be a proxy for deleterious childhood socio-economic conditions and environmental influences, including a lack of intellectual and cultural pursuits that have been shown to be associated with a higher risk of developing Alzheimer's disease. It may well be that the early life effects of 'using one's brain' persist over the life course.

Another possibility is that a high level of education may be a proxy for intelligence as more intelligent people are likely to obtain more formal education. The evidence that low intelligence may be linked with the development of dementia is quite varied. Lower pre-morbid intelligence has been found to predict the development of dementia in elderly people. More generally, lower pre-morbid intelligence predicts worse cognitive outcome following head injury. Possibly the most intriguing evidence, however, is from studies of older people that have access to early life measures of cognitive ability.

The 'Nun Study' involves a cohort of elderly Roman Catholic nuns who were assessed with a number having their brains studied post-mortem. Diary entries written in their late teenage years were examined for linguistic ability. Low linguistic ability during their teenage years was associated with Alzheimer's disease brain pathology at autopsy. One interpretation of these findings has been that incipient Alzheimer's disease was already present in the teenage nuns; certainly it has been shown that pathological changes of Alzheimer's disease may be present for 30 years before its clinical onset. Another interpretation is that the linguistic ability was a proxy for intelligence.[52]

A second study is based on the Scottish Mental Survey of 1932 in which almost every child at school in Scotland who was born in the calendar year 1921 took a group-administered mental ability test. These tests are stored in the University of Glasgow and have been transcribed onto a computer database. Researchers from the University of Edinburgh identified 173 persons with dementia from dementia case registers in Edinburgh that had completed the 1932 survey and compared them with persons without dementia who had completed the survey. They found that lower pre-morbid cognitive ability was associated with vascular dementia but not Alzheimer's disease.[53]

So how might intelligence reduce the risk of dementia? The Scottish study suggests that lower pre-morbid intelligence increases dementia risk through vascular disease. Perhaps those with less intelligence are prone to

making poor lifestyle choices regarding diet, smoking and exercise that increase their risk of vascular disease (see Chapter 3). This could be linked with the hypothesis that more intelligent people have a larger 'brain reserve'. The concept of brain reserve is based on the fact that our brains carry redundant neurons that act as a type of backup in times of need. In this hypothesis, when the brain is damaged, for example in a stroke or through the gradual development of Alzheimer's disease, the brain reserve comes into play to replace or cover for the damaged cells. If the brain reserve is inadequate to cover for the damage, the threshold of the disease is reached and the person becomes symptomatic. Thus, the larger the brain reserve, the greater the damage that can be sustained before symptoms occur. Whether this effect is due to there being 'further to fall' before reaching disease threshold, or whether the large brain reserve in some way resists the neuropathological changes, for example through greater cognitive flexibility, is unclear.[54] Whatever the model, a person with a large brain reserve may have incipient Alzheimer's disease for many years and be asymptomatic. In this situation, intelligence is delaying the onset of dementia.

Other important factors contribute to brain reserve including the previously described adverse childhood events. Any damage to the brain may reduce the reserve. For example, head injuries causing loss of consciousness for at least 15 minutes may increase the risk of Alzheimer's disease by up to twofold, though the studies are inconsistent and possibly the most methodologically sound prospective study had a negative result.[55] On the other hand, boxers may develop 'dementia pugilistica' due to repeated blows to the head. And recently controversy has arisen about American footballers being at increased risk of younger-onset dementia due to chronic traumatic encephalopathy from repeated concussions.[56] Jeff Astle, a former England football international, was found to have died from a degenerative brain disease due to 'heading' the football, a skill for which he was famous. Other types of previous brain damage including strokes and mental retardation may also increase the likelihood of dementia occurring.

Brain size is another factor – the larger the brain, the larger the brain reserve. This may be linked with intelligence as more intelligent people tend to have larger brains. People with larger brains, as measured by CT scans, MRI scans or head circumference, are less likely to develop the symptoms of Alzheimer's disease, even if they have the features of the disease in their brains at autopsy.

Mental activity

Mental activity also influences brain reserve. It is possible that mental activity enhances neuronal integrity through the action of better cerebral blood flow in reducing levels of stress and improving DNA repair. More tantalisingly, it may also enhance neuronal growth.[57] Numerous studies have shown that various forms of intellectual activity through life, even in the sixth and seventh decades, may protect against cognitive decline and enhance memory function. Hearing-impaired older people have been found to be at increased risk of dementia and one possible mechanism is lack of mental stimulation.[58]

Cognitive training is a formal therapy that aims to enhance cognitive function. It involves activities that focus on cognitive functions such as reasoning, memory and speed of information processing. One study, involving nearly 3000 participants in a six-week intervention, demonstrated that cognitive benefits lasted for up to five years and had some effect on everyday functioning.[59] A recent study from Chicago found that more frequent mental stimulation in old age led to better cognitive functioning over nearly five years.[60]

It may not just be the quantity of mental activity that is important. Deciding to stimulate your brain through a series of repetitive, boring mental exercises, or putting pressure on yourself by taking on an intellectual pursuit that is well beyond your capacity may be detrimental. Authors of memory books often recommend various mental exercises that include 'pegging' numbers to words for easier recall, visualising pictures with numbers and words, crossword puzzles, logic and graph puzzles, and exercises to improve the recall of word lists. Unless you enjoy doing these things it is unlikely to be of much benefit. Put simply, the mental activity should be fun!

Physical activity

People who are physically active often demonstrate less cognitive decline and a lower risk of dementia than those who are sedentary. There is also an association between midlife physical activity and late-life cognitive impairment.[61] There is convincing evidence that even short durations of aerobic exercise training can improve cognitive performance in normal older people and in persons at risk of Alzheimer's disease.[62] In those with dementia, physical exercise can slow the rate of cognitive decline. Interestingly, physical exercise undertaken in a social context appears to have the greatest benefit. Physical exercise can increase cerebral blood

flow and this may in turn be beneficial for mental function but this is unlikely to be the only way it might work as there is also evidence that people who exercise have higher levels of neurotrophic factors that are implicated in neurological repair. There are so many different reasons to embrace physical exercise it would not be surprising if it turns out that dementia prevention is another benefit. It has been estimated that physical inactivity might be responsible for nearly 13 per cent of Alzheimer's disease cases worldwide and perhaps as many as 21 per cent of cases in the US. A 10 per cent reduction of physical inactivity worldwide could potentially prevent 380,000 Alzheimer's disease cases.[63]

The implication of these findings are that mental and physical activities throughout life may continue to impart a protective role especially if there is an element of social contact as well.

Summary

Traditional strategies to prevent disease have focused upon disease elimination. In the case of dementia, a delay in the onset of the disease may have a preventive effect as potential victims may die of other disorders before they develop dementia. An understanding of risk and protective factors for dementia is required before any preventive strategies can be undertaken. Universal prevention strategies are those that can be applied to the whole population and often involve lifestyle changes including those related to diet, exercise, mental activity and social participation.

Table 2.2 summarises the various universal dementia prevention strategies and comments on the strength of evidence and potential tolerability. Most universal strategies are easy to apply and have a wide range of health benefits and few drawbacks. Examples include dietary changes to improve antioxidants in our food, continuing physical exercise and education. The extent to which these strategies may reduce the risk of dementia is unclear but they are unlikely to harm.

Table 2.2 Universal dementia prevention strategies

Risk factor	Prevention strategy	Strength of evidence 0 = no evidence 1 = weak 2 = modest 3 = strong 4 = proven	Tolerability 0 = intolerable 1 = low 2 = moderate 3 = very tolerable
Age oxidative metabolism (the breakdown of nutrients that yield energy in the presence of oxygen)	Antioxidants – vitamins C and E-rich foods (not supplements) Antioxidants – folate rich foods, possibly supplements	2 – controlled trials equivocal, could delay dementia onset 2 – controlled trials equivocal, may reduce the risk of cognitive decline	3 – unlikely to harm and likely to have other health benefits 3 – unlikely to harm and likely to have other health benefits
Dietary pattern	Mediterranean Diet	2 – controlled trials equivocal for dementia prevention but may improve cognition	3 – unlikely to harm and likely to have other health benefits
Brain reserve	Life-long education, aerobic physical exercise, mental and social activity	3 – mounting evidence in controlled trials of cognitive benefits in persons with and without dementia	3 – unlikely to harm and likely to have other health benefits

Prevention of Dementia

Strategies for Individuals at Increased Risk

In Chapter 2, prevention strategies that are applicable to everybody were considered. In this chapter, strategies that are applicable either to individuals at increased risk of dementia or to individuals already experiencing mild symptoms of possible dementia (mild cognitive impairment) are considered.

Selective dementia prevention strategies

Selective prevention strategies are directed towards individuals because they have established risk factors for a disease. Common examples include weight reduction in overweight people to reduce the risk of coronary artery disease and diabetes, smoking cessation to reduce the risk of lung, heart and blood vessel disease, and increased calcium intake in people with osteoporosis to reduce the risk of fractures. Some dementia prevention strategies that are in this category may be useful for everybody and not just those with risk factors of dementia and I indicate those that are most promising. Not all established dementia risk factors currently have effective preventive strategies.

Genetic factors

Genetic factors are causative in many younger-onset (pre-senile) dementias but there is now mounting evidence that they also contribute in a major way to the development of late-onset Alzheimer's disease. Genetic factors and age are the two main established risk factors for Alzheimer's disease. Unfortunately, there are currently no recognised preventive strategies that can directly reduce the genetic risk.

Recently, however, a rare mutation on the amyloid precursor protein (APP) gene that reduces the risk of Alzheimer's disease was reported in *Nature*. The research from Iceland indicated that Icelanders who carry the mutation are more than five times more likely to reach 85 without being diagnosed with Alzheimer's disease compared with those who lack it. There was also a lower risk of cognitive decline that was not due to Alzheimer's disease.[1] This provides a model for drug development as a drug that mimics this effect could potentially slow cognitive decline and prevent Alzheimer's disease.

Familial Alzheimer's disease

Most of the highly publicised advances in the genetics of Alzheimer's disease have come from the study of very rare families with familial Alzheimer's disease (FAD) that account for 2 to 5 per cent of cases of Alzheimer's disease. FAD is an autosomal dominant disease, which means that 50 per cent of each generation develop Alzheimer's disease, usually between the ages of 40 and 60 years. Causative mutations on chromosome 14 (presenilin-1 gene), chromosome 1 (presenilin-2 gene) and chromosome 21 (APP gene) have been found in these families. Hints that chromosome 21 could be implicated came with the finding that there was a higher rate of Down syndrome, a genetic disorder due to abnormalities on chromosome 21, in the family history of Alzheimer patients, and with the observation that the majority of persons with Down syndrome who survive to late adulthood develop dementia.[2]

In individuals with younger-onset Alzheimer's disease, diagnostic DNA testing will confirm whether it is a familial form, although in 30 per cent of cases no mutation will be found. Predictive testing of family members can then be undertaken, if desired, to determine which individuals have the mutation and allow for genetic counselling. Currently, there are no specific treatments available for these family members, and in the absence of such treatment, the take-up for predictive testing is low.[3] The potential for gene-modifying therapies is discussed in Chapter 13.

Late-onset Alzheimer's disease

The vast majority of cases of Alzheimer's disease are not due to a mutation in a single gene, but are due to polymorphisms, which are where the presence of a number of genetic risk factors interact with environmental factors. Inheritance in this type of genetics does not follow simple rules that allow for neat predictions of chance. When relatives of

patients diagnosed with Alzheimer's disease ask what their chances are of getting Alzheimer's disease, the question is not easily answered. The longer we live the more likely we are to develop dementia; by the age of 100 most people are likely to have dementia. If we consider only the first-degree relatives of people who develop Alzheimer's disease by the age of 85 years, there is a threefold to fourfold increased risk of their developing Alzheimer's disease, as compared to the general community. This translates to a lifetime risk of between 16 and 20 per cent, which may be quite worrying. In considering this risk, however, it is necessary to take into account the likelihood of a person surviving to a certain age. Using actuarial tables in combination with these risk percentages, it has been calculated, for example, that a first-degree relative of a person with Alzheimer's disease surviving to the age of 78 years has less than 10 per cent chance of having developed Alzheimer's disease. Overall, less than one third of the risk is realised in the normal lifespan.[4] Putting it in these terms reassures many relatives, particularly those who are concerned that they may develop Alzheimer's disease at a younger age, which can be shown by similar calculations to be an extremely rare event. For second-degree relatives such as grandchildren, the risk of developing Alzheimer's disease is probably less than twice the overall population risk, though there has been only limited research on this to date.

Only one gene, that for apolipoprotein E (APOE), has been definitely associated with late-onset Alzheimer's disease. Apolipoprotein E, a protein synthesised in the liver and brain, is involved in lipid metabolism and tissue repair. There are three common alleles (forms) of the APOE gene, known as APOE ε2, APOE ε3 and APOE ε4, which are on chromosome 19. In 1993, it was observed that the frequency of APOE ε4 in patients with Alzheimer's disease was greater than that found in age-matched controls. This has been confirmed in numerous studies around the world. Further, the risk is higher in people who are homozygous for APOE ε4 (that is, have two APOE ε4 genes – one inherited from each parent) than in those who are heterozygous (only one APOE ε4 gene). These findings suggest that APOE ε4 status increases the risk of developing Alzheimer's disease, but the mechanism is as yet unknown.

Current opinion is that APOE ε4 is a susceptibility gene being neither necessary nor sufficient for Alzheimer's disease development. The APOE ε4 genotype determines when rather than whether a person develops Alzheimer's disease. Carriers of APOE ε4 appear to develop Alzheimer's disease earlier, with estimates suggesting that, at most, some

50 per cent of people who are homozygous for APOE ε4 will develop Alzheimer's disease within their lifetime. Overall approximately 15 to 20 per cent of Alzheimer cases are attributable to APOE ε4. A review of the interaction of APOE ε4 with other risk factors for Alzheimer's disease found that APOE ε4 increases the risk of dementia when associated with greater fat consumption, particularly saturated fats.[5] There is also some suggestion that carriers of the APOE ε2 gene may have some protection from getting Alzheimer's disease and this has been supported by the high rates found in centenarians.

Consensus statements from Alzheimer's Disease International and Alzheimer's Association and the National Institute of Aging in the US have concluded that there is no current role for APOE genotyping in the prediction of risk of developing Alzheimer's disease.[6] While the presence of the APOE ε4 gene may increase accuracy in diagnosing Alzheimer's disease in persons with dementia, its absence has little value in endorsing or refuting the diagnosis. Of course, a better understanding of how the APOE ε4 protein influences the pathophysiology of Alzheimer's disease may result in potential preventive strategies that target APOE.

Frontotemporal dementia

Around 10 to 15 per cent of people with frontotemporal dementia have a familial form.[7] In 1998 it was discovered that a mutation in the microtubule-associated protein tau (MAPT) gene linked to chromosome 17 causes a form of frontotemporal dementia called frontotemporal dementia with parkinsonism (FTDP-17). Other mutations on chromosome 17 have been subsequently discovered that cause a range of MAPT-related tauopathies including FTDP-17, progressive supranuclear palsy, corticobasal degeneration, mild late-onset parkinsonism, and dementia with epilepsy.[8] In each case there is autosomal dominant inheritance which means that there is a 50 per cent chance that a child will inherit the condition.

There is also some overlap with motor neurone disease in this spectrum as frontotemporal dementia and motor neurone disease are related. In 2011 two international groups of investigators independently discovered a mutation of the C9ORF72 gene on chromosome 9 that may account for around 12 per cent of familial frontotemporal dementia, and as much as 22 per cent of familial motor neurone disease.[9, 10] It is currently unclear how this mutation leads to either disease.

Vascular dementia

Cerebral autosomal dominant arteriopathy with subcortical infarcts and leukoencephalopathy (CADASIL) is a rare autosomal dominant form of younger-onset vascular dementia that usually commences from age 30–60. Characteristically there is a history of migraine with aura, transient ischaemic attacks (mini strokes), mood disturbances, apathy and cerebrovascular disease as noted by diffuse white matter lesions and subcortical infarcts on brain scans. Mutations are found on the NOTCH3 gene in over 95 per cent of cases.[11]

Vascular risk factors

It has long been recognised that factors that increase the risk of stroke – the so-called vascular risk factors – will also increase the risk of vascular dementia. Vascular risk factors include hypertension (high blood pressure), smoking, obesity, diabetes, high cholesterol and low-density lipoproteins. The effects of each factor appears to be additive – that is, the more factors that are present the higher the risk of dementia.[12] Similarly the metabolic syndrome, which is a clustering of disorders that include abdominal obesity, high triglycerides, low high-density lipoprotein levels, hypertension and/or high blood sugar is associated with increased risk of cognitive impairment.[13]

What has been surprising is the discovery that these factors also increase the risk of Alzheimer's disease. One of the reasons for this might be that Alzheimer's disease and vascular dementia could share common genetic factors and there is also the recognition that most people with Alzheimer's disease have some degree of vascular damage in the brain as well. Many vascular risk factors can be modified by simple lifestyle changes but despite this there has been little research that has directly examined their preventive potential.

Hypertension

High blood pressure is probably the single most important risk factor for stroke and vascular dementia. This is certainly the case in midlife where a history of high blood pressure in combination with heart disease or diabetes increases the risk of vascular dementia by up to sixfold and also Alzheimer's disease by two-to-threefold.[14] It has been estimated that worldwide about 5 per cent of Alzheimer's disease cases are potentially attributable to midlife hypertension and perhaps as much as 8 per cent

of cases in the US.[15] To date there have been no studies of the midlife treatment of hypertension to see whether effective treatment reduces the risk of dementia in late life, but if it were effective, a 10 per cent reduction of midlife hypertension prevalence would result in 160,000 fewer Alzheimer's disease cases worldwide.[16]

In late life, the association between hypertension and dementia is more controversial with some studies showing an association and others not; some suggest that while hypertension is a risk factor for dementia, blood pressure may decrease three to six years before its onset. Similarly, treatment of hypertension in late life has had mixed results with only two out of five trials showing a reduction in dementia cases. Of the two positive studies, the Syst-Eur trial demonstrated a 50 per cent reduction in cases of dementia, mainly Alzheimer's disease, after two years of treatment on antihypertensive medication. Extrapolating from this study, over five years, the treatment of 1000 hypertensive people would prevent 19 cases of dementia.[17] The other trial, the PROGRESS study, involved treatment on antihypertensive therapy alone or in combination with diuretic medication or placebo and it followed up this treatment for four years. While there was a 12 per cent reduction in cases of dementia, this was largely related to vascular cases, which was in keeping with the overall reduction in stroke by up to 43 per cent depending on the regimen used.[18]

These findings indicate that optimal treatment of high blood pressure is likely to be an important preventive measure for dementia, though the degree of specificity for any particular type of dementia remains uncertain. Whether specific types of antihypertensive medication, such as calcium channel blockers and angiotensin-converting enzyme inhibitors, are more effective than others and whether the cognitive benefits are brought about by mechanisms other than lowering blood pressure is uncertain. It is also unclear whether similar benefits can be obtained by other lifestyle measures that are known to reduce high blood pressure and improve health, such as reducing salt in the diet, weight control, physical fitness and optimal alcohol intake. Common sense would suggest that these should form the cornerstone of a lifestyle intended to reduce the risk of dementia.[19, 20, 21]

Smoking

Smoking is strongly associated with cardiovascular disease, peripheral vascular disease, stroke and vascular dementia. For some years, studies appeared to suggest that smoking had a mild protective effect against Alzheimer's disease, possibly from the nicotine, but larger, better-quality

studies have shown that smoking is associated with up to double the risk of Alzheimer's disease.[22] Indeed, it has been estimated that nearly 14 per cent of Alzheimer's disease cases worldwide are potentially attributable to smoking.[23] The relationship may not be as simple as it appears at first glance however, because smoking appears to interact with other risk factors including alcohol, gender and genetic factors to both increase and decrease the chances of getting Alzheimer's disease. More research is needed to tease out what may be happening.

At this stage, however, encouraging older people to stop smoking should be considered as part of a strategy to reduce the incidence of cognitive impairment. A 10 per cent reduction in smoking prevalence worldwide could potentially lower the prevalence of Alzheimer's disease by about 412,000 cases.[24] Another consumer warning that could be placed on cigarette packets might be 'Remember to stop smoking to remember'. There are many reasons to stop smoking – and dementia risk is yet another.

Diabetes mellitus

Diabetes mellitus is associated with moderate cognitive deficits and brain changes that may be referred to as diabetic encephalopathy.[25] Recent studies have shown that type 2 diabetes, which usually develops in mid-to-late life and is believed to be strongly influenced by diet and obesity, increases the risk of Alzheimer's disease by around one-and-a-half to twofold and vascular dementia by over twofold. There might be interactions with the APOE gene but research findings are inconsistent.[26] Both vascular and non-vascular factors are likely to play a role in dementia in diabetes, where mixed aetiology is likely. Approximately 2 per cent of Alzheimer's disease cases worldwide are possibly attributable to diabetes, perhaps a higher proportion in western countries, with a 10 per cent reduction in diabetes worldwide estimated to potentially reduce the number of cases by over 80,000.[27] There are no high quality studies that have examined whether better diabetic control improves cognition and reduces dementia risk. Drugs used to treat diabetes, such as rosiglitazone, have been investigated as treatments for Alzheimer's disease but were found to be ineffective.

Cholesterol

There are a number of links between cholesterol and Alzheimer's disease. Major studies have shown that people who have cholesterol levels above 6.5 in midlife increase their risk of Alzheimer's disease in later life by at least two-and-a-half-fold.[28] In later life the relationship between

cholesterol levels and Alzheimer's disease is less clear, with some suggestion that cholesterol levels decline some years before the onset of dementia, mirroring the pattern noted earlier with blood pressure.[29] There is a convergence of research, as the previously mentioned apolipoprotein E, which is associated with an individual's risk of developing Alzheimer's disease, carries cholesterol in the brain. It also promotes the formation of amyloid plaques that are a hallmark of Alzheimer pathology. There is also some laboratory research that suggests that high levels of cholesterol cause the body to produce more amyloid precursor protein and hence more beta-amyloid.[30]

There have been attempts to reduce dementia risk by lowering cholesterol levels. Statins are a class of drugs that lower levels of low-density lipoprotein (LDL) cholesterol – the type most strongly linked with coronary artery disease and stroke – by blocking a liver enzyme essential for cholesterol production. Examples include fluvastatin, simvastatin, atorvastatin and pravastatin. While statins reduce the risk of stroke by 29 per cent, findings from randomised controlled trials have been inconsistent about their role in reducing the risk of dementia.[31, 32]

There is evidence that cholesterol metabolism plays a role in the development of Alzheimer's disease, although its relative importance in the overall picture remains unclear. Another aspect that requires further attention is whether cholesterol levels currently regarded as normal are in fact potentially harmful. In other words, are there potential benefits in lowering everyone's cholesterol level, not just those whose levels are high?

Obesity – high Body Mass Index and high calorie intake
Obesity and high Body Mass Index (BMI) in midlife, and possibly late life, are associated with an increased risk of developing dementia, although similar to the situation with blood pressure and cholesterol there appears to be a reduction in BMI before the onset of dementia.[33] One Swedish study found that for every 1.0 increase in BMI at age 70 years in women (but not men!) the risk of Alzheimer's disease increased by 36 per cent.[34] One report found that individuals who eat a high-calorie diet (more than 1870 kilocalories per day) with high saturated fats have more than double the risk of Alzheimer's disease, but only if they are a carrier of the APOE ε4 gene. Non-carriers of the APOE ε4 gene were not at increased risk with such a diet.[35] This is another good example of the importance of the interaction between genetic and lifestyle risk factors.

Midlife obesity has been estimated to be responsible for about 2 per cent of cases of Alzheimer's disease worldwide, but in the US with its

obesity epidemic, it might account for over 7 per cent of cases. A 10 per cent reduction of midlife obesity worldwide could potentially prevent 67,000 Alzheimer's disease cases.[36]

Atherosclerosis and reduced cerebral blood flow

It is probably self-evident that a reduction in blood flow to the brain will adversely affect brain function. It is well known that blockage of the main arteries to the brain can result in strokes and hence vascular dementia. More subtle reductions in cerebral blood flow that occur in people with cardiovascular and other circulatory problems might also be damaging. Atherosclerosis (hardening of the arteries) damages the carotid and vertebrobasilar arteries, the main blood vessels supplying the brain. This results in a build-up of platelets, blocking the arteries and acting as a source for small blood clots (emboli) to pepper the brain. Atrial fibrillation, in which there is an irregular heart rate, can have the same effect. These frequently result in transient ischaemic attacks (TIAs). For many years, low-dose aspirin has been prescribed due to its ability to stop platelets from sticking together and has been shown to reduce the risk of stroke and TIAs. There is contradictory evidence about aspirin slowing the progression of dementia and no studies have found that aspirin prevents dementia, but a recent Swedish study found that low-dose aspirin slowed cognitive decline over five years in older women at high cardiovascular risk.[37] As aspirin is a potent cause of stomach irritation and bleeding, unless other vascular risk factors demand its use to reduce the risk of stroke, it cannot be recommended as a routine preventive measure for dementia.

Coronary artery bypass surgery

Between 50 and 80 per cent of patients undergoing coronary artery bypass surgery become confused after the surgery and have cognitive impairment at discharge from hospital. While many have questioned the importance of this cognitive deterioration, there is now mounting evidence that impairments are still found in 42 per cent of patients five years after surgery.[38] Because persistent cognitive impairments are associated with early post-operative confusion, efforts to reduce post-operative confusion may prevent such impairments. Pre-operative cognitive impairment is well established as a major risk factor for post-operative confusion with about 35 per cent of patients undergoing coronary artery bypass surgery being cognitively impaired before surgery.[39] This should not be too

surprising as most of these patients have multiple vascular risk factors as previously described. However, it is unclear whether the actual coronary bypass surgery predisposes to dementia and further research is required to determine if this is the case.

Gender – the role of hormone replacement therapy

While there does not appear to be an overall difference in the rates of dementia between men and women, there are differences in individual types of dementia. Some studies show that women have slightly higher rates of Alzheimer's disease and that men have higher rates of vascular dementia.

The higher rate of Alzheimer's disease in women may relate to a combination of increased longevity, increased survival with the disease, and some increase in intrinsic vulnerability. The latter may link with evidence that oestrogen protects the brain from damage, possibly by regulating nerve growth. It has been observed that women who are taking oestrogen as Hormone Replacement Therapy (HRT) after the menopause have approximately a 30 per cent lower risk of developing Alzheimer's disease, particularly if they have been taking it for at least ten years.[40] As these studies were not designed specifically to determine whether HRT might prevent dementia, a number of other risk factors for dementia related to lifestyle and education were not controlled for and so it could be that these other factors explain the difference.

Large trials in the US, Europe and Australasia designed to address this issue were halted due to safety concerns. The Women's Health Initiative Study involving 16,600 women taking a combination of oestrogen and progesterone, which was due to be completed in 2005, was abruptly halted in July 2002 as a 26 per cent increase in breast cancer, and higher rates of heart disease, stroke and blood clots, were recorded after 5.2 years of treatment. Even the risk of dementia was increased. The researchers found that the risks were outweighing the benefits.[41] Within days an expert committee from the Australian Therapeutic Goods Administration recommended that combined HRT not be used in long-term replacement. The cessation of the Women's Health Initiative Study had a flow-on effect to other studies with the Women's International Study of long Duration Oestrogen after Menopause – Cognition (WISDOM–COG) being halted after only one year of a proposed ten-year study with similar findings.[42] The Women's Health Initiative Memory Study examined the effects of oestrogen therapy alone in post-menopausal women and found it was

ineffective in preventing dementia or mild cognitive impairment and in fact increased the risk of cognitive impairment.[43]

Several trials of oestrogen in the treatment of women with Alzheimer's disease have been negative, but this may simply mean that the oestrogen was given too late. The pros and cons of oestrogen-only HRT are still heavily debated as there is concern that the type of oestrogen used in the halted studies (conjugated equine oestrogen) may have more deleterious cognitive effects than oestradiol that has most commonly been used in the epidemiological studies. There is also concern that the HRT may have been commenced too late (age 65 years and over) for cognitive benefits.[44] The other benefits of oestrogen-only HRT include an overall 44 per cent reduction in mortality over five years and up to 50 per cent reduction in hip fractures, against the previously mentioned concerns about increased risk of breast cancer and deep vein thrombosis.[45] For post-menopausal women, any decision to use HRT should only be made after carefully considering these potential risks and benefits; at this stage there is insufficient evidence to support its routine use for the prevention of Alzheimer's disease alone.

The increased risk of vascular dementia in men has mainly been attributed to lifestyle factors that men are more likely to engage in rather than any inherent male factor, although there is evidence that androgens may increase the risk of cardiac disease so there may be indirect effects. Some research has found that older men with higher levels of free testosterone had better memory and cognitive function. This may mean that testosterone could play a protective role against cognitive decline but this idea is speculative.[46]

Inflammation – the role of anti-inflammatory medication

Both Alzheimer's disease and vascular dementia are characterised by inflammatory responses that are believed to contribute to the death of nerve cells. Epidemiological studies have identified a reduced risk of Alzheimer's disease in people with arthritis and leprosy being treated with anti-inflammatory drugs. Longitudinal studies have shown that the consumption of anti-inflammatory medications for two or more years reduces the risk of Alzheimer's disease by up to 80 per cent, but has no effect on the risk of vascular dementia.[47]

In contrast, treatment studies of Alzheimer patients with low-dose steroids (prednisone) and two non-steroidal anti-inflammatory drugs (NSAIDs) – celecoxib and indomethacin – have failed to demonstrate a

significant effect. It is possible that the dose of prednisone was too low to be beneficial and there are also concerns that to be effective, anti-inflammatory medication may need to be given very early in the course of the disease, possibly before the individual is symptomatic. The Alzheimer's Disease Anti-inflammatory Prevention Trial (the ADAPT study) was designed to test this with the NSAIDs celecoxib and naproxen. The study was due to run over seven years but was terminated early due to safety concerns. At termination after a mean of two years the treatment groups showed trends for increased risks of Alzheimer's disease. The investigators continued to monitor the participants for another two years after treatment cessation and found that increased risk of dementia remained notable for two and a half years, especially in the participants with cognitive impairment at time of enrolment. However, after two to three years a reduction in incidence of Alzheimer's disease was found in participants treated with naproxen and no cognitive impairment at the time of enrolment, a finding mirrored in cerebrospinal fluid (CSF) findings suggestive of reduced Alzheimer-type neurodegeneration.[48]

These findings indicate that NSAIDs may be deleterious in later stages of the pathogenesis of Alzheimer's disease and that treatment would need to begin in asymptomatic individuals with benefits emerging after a few years.[49] This is consistent with the epidemiological studies that tend to show no benefit in use in the two years before onset of dementia. Further studies are required to determine how long NSAIDs would need to be used for and how long the benefit might last.

As these medications have many side effects including stomach irritation, bleeding and anaemia, they cannot be recommended for prevention of Alzheimer's disease until further sound placebo-controlled studies have been published.

Occupational and chemical exposures

The search for occupational risk factors for dementia has generally yielded disappointing results. The large French PAQUID study (personnes agees quid) did not find any occupational risk factors for Alzheimer's disease. Several follow-up studies have suggested that occupational exposure to extremely low frequency electromagnetic fields is related to an increased risk of dementia and Alzheimer's disease. These occupations, including electricians, machinists, carpenters, sheet metal workers, toolmakers, seamstresses, typists and welders, involve the use of electric motors close to the body. Better shielding of electric motors might have a protective

effect. Linkage of exposure to extremely low frequency electromagnetic fields and Alzheimer's disease has biological plausibility.[50]

One Canadian study has found that occupational exposure to fumigants/defoliants increased the risk of Alzheimer's disease by over fourfold. This is biologically plausible as the chemicals have an adverse effect on neuronal activity.[51] Another study in the agricultural community in Cache County, Utah, found occupational exposure to organophosphate pesticides to be associated with increased risk of dementia and Alzheimer's disease in late life.[52] Better protective clothing in the handling of these chemicals might have a role in reducing dementia.

There has been some evidence that people in less mentally demanding jobs are more likely to get Alzheimer's disease in later life. Some studies have found higher numbers of manual workers have dementia than would be expected by chance, suggesting the possibility of occupational exposure,[53, 54] but others have not confirmed the findings.[55] It is more likely, however, that these findings are confounded by factors such as education and lifestyle.

Anaesthesia

There is evidence from animal models that inhaled anaesthetic exposure increases pathology associated with Alzheimer's disease. Studies of the effects of exposure to anaesthetics in humans have shown conflicting results regarding the later development of Alzheimer's disease. Post-operative cognitive decline is well described but the long-term outcome is unclear. Many caregivers anecdotally report that after such an episode their loved ones fail to regain their previous level of cognitive function. An anaesthetics consensus statement concluded that there is sufficient evidence to warrant further investigation with more definitive research.[56]

Delirium (acute confusional state)

Older hospitalised people are at high risk of developing delirium, otherwise known as an acute confusional state. In most cases there are identifiable medical causes – infections, reduced brain blood supply, side effects of medication, dehydration and recent surgery, to name a few. While delirium is a sign of severe illness and is associated with increased mortality, treatment of the underlying causes usually results in recovery of mental function, although symptoms might persist for months. Dementia is a risk factor for delirium and it is well established that when persons

with dementia become ill, their confusion increases. This has recently been quantified in a study in which persons with Alzheimer's disease that had an episode of delirium declined three times faster than those that did not.[57]

There is some evidence that people without dementia who become delirious have an increased risk of developing dementia. Some do not fully recover, others recover only to decline in the following few years. Although the most likely explanation is that incipient dementia was present at the time of hospitalisation and the delirium represented a breach of symptom threshold, there is a possibility that delirium may cause permanent brain damage. One recent study from Norway found that in hip fracture patients without dementia pre-fracture, post-operative delirium was the main predictor for the development of dementia 6 months later.[58]

It is unclear whether strategies to prevent delirium could be regarded as selective strategies for high-risk individuals or indicated strategies for individuals with early symptoms. Sharon Inouye, from Yale University, has demonstrated in a series of elegant studies that the rate of delirium can be reduced in the hospitalised elderly by a combination of strategies that include early identification of high-risk individuals, rehydration, reality orientation, mobilisation and mental stimulation. It is not known whether this intervention will prevent dementia.[59]

Indicated dementia prevention strategies

Indicated prevention strategies target individuals who are showing early symptoms of disease but may not reach full criteria for the disease, or are not showing any damage from the disease. Common examples include coronary artery bypass surgery to treat mild angina so that heart attacks are prevented, excision of pre-malignant skin lesions, and removal of pre-cancerous bowel polyps. Currently there are no proven strategies that prevent the progression of early symptoms of mild cognitive impairment to dementia.

Mild cognitive impairment

Many terms have been used to describe states of mild cognitive disturbance that are not severe enough to qualify for the diagnosis of dementia. These include 'mild cognitive impairment', 'age-associated memory impairment' and 'benign senescent forgetfulness'. Each is defined in slightly different ways and each is associated with an increased risk of developing dementia.

Mild cognitive impairment (MCI) has received most attention recently and is described in more detail in Chapter 4.

Persons with MCI diagnosed in a memory clinic will progress to Alzheimer's disease at a rate of 10 to 15 per cent per year, compared with healthy control subjects who convert at a rate of 1 to 2 per cent per year.[60] A research group at the Mayo Clinic in the US has been observing a group of subjects with MCI for more than ten years and has demonstrated a conversion to Alzheimer's disease of up to 80 per cent, with another 10 per cent reverting to normal.[61] Survival rates for MCI subjects over a seven-year period are midway between those of normal elderly people and Alzheimer's patients. Although therapies are being developed that might prevent progression of MCI to Alzheimer's disease, there is no evidence to support prescribing therapeutic agents.

This research highlights one of the key ethical issues in this area. Defining MCI as a pathological state has opened the door to the pharmaceutical industry to develop agents to treat it; the industry is thus becoming a driving force to maintain MCI as a diagnostic entity. Critics of the current application of the MCI concept believe there is still insufficient evidence to warrant this distinction from the other age-related cognitive changes previously described. It is not that it is doubted that such states exist, only that their current identification is too imprecise. In recognition of this quandary, the new research diagnostic criteria for pre-clinical Alzheimer's disease incorporate the use of biomarkers, thus allowing for more accurate identification of those individuals with MCI that have prodromal Alzheimer's disease and facilitating drug trials aimed to prevent progression of pre-clinical Alzheimer's disease to clinical Alzheimer's disease.[62] The new diagnostic criteria, new treatments and biomarkers are discussed in more detail in Chapter 13.

Another issue highlighted by this dilemma is the prospect that while a successful treatment for a person with MCI may be defined as non-progression to Alzheimer's disease, it may not result in any meaningful improvement in the individual's memory and so may result in the person spending more time living with a significant disability.

Depression, stress and anxiety

Prospective studies of whether depression may be aetiologically linked to cognitive decline and dementia have yielded variable results. Statistical analysis of pooled data has found that depression was associated with

an increased risk of subsequent dementia. It has been estimated that about 10 per cent of Alzheimer's disease cases worldwide are potentially attributable to depression.[63] Older people with depression have a twofold to threefold risk of developing dementia – but it is quite possible that their depression is part of the evolving dementia, particularly Alzheimer's disease, which may not become apparent for a few years.[64] Depression in early to mid adulthood has been found to be associated with an increased risk of vascular dementia, but not Alzheimer's disease.[65, 66] This may be mediated by vascular risk factors. There is no evidence that effective treatment of depression alters any of the dementia risk. A 10 per cent reduction in depression prevalence, however, could potentially result in a reduction of 326,000 Alzheimer's cases worldwide.[67]

Many wonder whether stress and anxiety can cause dementia. Until recently there has been little research that has demonstrated a link. Certainly in much the same way as with depression, anxiety symptoms are common in the early stages of evolving cognitive impairment, but in this situation are not likely to be the cause of the dementia. Indeed one study that recently reported a link between benzodiazepine use (drugs such as diazepam used to treat anxiety) and dementia was perhaps demonstrating this.[68] There is also the evidence discussed in Chapter 2 about the possible role that childhood adversity might have in predisposing to dementia, and certainly there is stronger evidence linking childhood adversity with anxiety and depression in adulthood.[69]

Post-traumatic stress disorder (PTSD) is a severe manifestation of anxiety and stress occurring in individuals that have had exposure to major trauma such as happens in war or natural disasters. Two recent studies of PTSD in Vietnam war veterans in the US have demonstrated an almost double risk of dementia in war veterans with PTSD even when other factors were taken into account.[70, 71] A systematic review of studies that have examined the effect of PTSD on cognition concluded that individuals with PTSD, particularly veterans, show signs of cognitive impairment when tested with neuropsychological instruments, more so than individuals exposed to trauma who do not have PTSD.[72] These studies do not prove that PTSD causes dementia but certainly detect an association that requires further research.

Some unproven factors and treatments

Over the years there have been many factors that have been suggested as potential 'causes' of dementia and Alzheimer's disease in particular or as treatments to prevent dementia but research has failed to substantiate the claims. Here I mention some of the prominent ones.

Aluminium

Since the 1960s there have been repeated claims that aluminium may be important in the development of dementia. Aluminium is known to be toxic to the nervous system. Many years ago, chronic renal dialysis patients developed 'dialysis dementia' due to high levels of aluminium that accumulated during the dialysis process, a situation that no longer occurs. Further, there was some evidence of increased levels of aluminium in the brains of persons with Alzheimer's disease, and some animal studies found that high levels of aluminium may provoke Alzheimer's-type changes in the brain. These claims led to many people throwing out all of their aluminium cooking utensils. However, numerous epidemiological studies have failed to demonstrate any consistent association between levels of aluminium in diet, water or medication (antacids) and Alzheimer's disease. In addition, the pathological changes found in the brains of 'dialysis dementia' patients are quite different from Alzheimer's disease. So aluminium seems an unlikely factor at this point.

Viral infections

Viruses are implicated in so many diseases that it is not surprising they have been considered as potential factors in Alzheimer's disease. The discovery of the HIV virus, and its ability to cause dementia many years later, added impetus to the search. Other viruses, such as the herpes zoster virus that causes shingles, are sequestered in nerve cells for decades after initial exposure before becoming symptomatic. This means that viral exposure in childhood, or possibly *in utero*, could theoretically be involved. So far research has been largely negative, though one study did find higher rates of herpes simplex infection in Alzheimer patients. Much stronger evidence is required before any concerns should be expressed.

Food-borne toxins

Several rare neurological conditions have been linked with the intake of food-borne toxins found in legumes in Africa, India and Guam. In Canada, an outbreak of a neurological disorder similar to Alzheimer's

disease occurred among people who had eaten mussels contaminated with demoic acid. These examples provide evidence that food-borne toxins could potentially be implicated in Alzheimer's disease but no specific toxins have been identified that affect the broader population.

Bacterial infection

Researchers from Washington University, St Louis in the US have discovered that common bacteria responsible for urinary infections, wound infections and food poisoning (Escherichia coli and salmonella) can sometimes produce amyloid protein which increases their resistance to antibiotics.[73] This raises the question as to whether bacteria may play a role in amyloid production in the brain. Much more research is required.

Ginkgo biloba

The Chinese herb ginkgo biloba is thought to increase circulation to the brain. In Europe and some Asian countries, standardised extracts from ginkgo leaves are taken to treat a wide range of symptoms, including dizziness, inflammation, and reduced blood flow to the brain and other areas of impaired circulation. It is routinely prescribed in Europe for memory problems and although there is some evidence that it may be beneficial, the studies are not strong. Two studies funded in the US by the National Institute on Aging and the National Center for Complementary and Alternative Medicine reported their combined findings on over 3000 older adults at risk of dementia who took 240mg of ginkgo biloba or a placebo for an average of about six years. They did not find any effect in reducing the overall incidence of dementia or Alzheimer's disease in normal individuals or in those with mild cognitive impairment.[74] Recently a third large study from France had similar findings.[75] Thus there is no evidence to recommend its use for preventing dementia, particularly as ginkgo can cause stomach bleeding, especially when taken with aspirin.

Summary

Although there are now numerous factors that have been identified that increase the risk of dementia, it is fair to say that the factors that have the strongest impact are currently the hardest to change – age and genes. This is emphasised by research that has shown that persons with superior health over the age of 85 years are not protected from developing Alzheimer's disease. In the case of Alzheimer's disease, altering most of

the other factors may delay the onset of dementia rather than eliminate it, though attention to vascular risk factors and lifestyle offers better hope of elimination of vascular dementia. Delay of onset may be as good as cure, but it is possible that the general health benefits will also delay other potentially terminal diseases in old age as well.

In Table 3.1 I summarise the various selective and indicated prevention strategies, comment on the strength of evidence for each and their potential tolerability. Some strategies are easy to apply and have a wide range of health benefits and few, if any, drawbacks. Other strategies, such as anti-inflammatory medications and hormone replacement therapy, may have potentially greater effect but are currently unproven and have significant adverse effects. In between are strategies that are indicated in specific circumstances, like high blood pressure and cholesterol, where the treatments may have adverse effects and their potential to prevent dementia is not entirely proven. As there are new studies published regularly in this field, you should consult your doctor for specific advice.

The great appeal of substances such as ginkgo biloba and vitamins is that they are not prescription drugs. They are also relatively cheap and easily available. However, little is known about the side effects of supplements taken in large doses over a prolonged period, and there is some evidence that supplements do not work in the same way as naturally occurring vitamins in food. The consumer should be cautious in their use.

We are on the cusp of dementia prevention that may have some meaningful outcomes; future prospects are discussed in Chapter 13.

Table 3.1 Selective and indicated dementia prevention strategies

Risk factor	Prevention strategy	Strength of evidence 0 = no evidence 1 = weak 2 = modest 3 = strong 4 = proven	Tolerability 0 = intolerable 1 = low 2 = moderate 3 = very tolerable
		1. Selective strategies – people at high risk	
Gender – oestrogen deficiency in women	Hormone replacement therapy in post-menopausal women	1 – needs placebo-controlled prospective trials, only 30% risk reduction	1 – other health benefits are currently a stronger indication and there are adverse effects
Inflammation – early effects of AD	Anti-inflammatory medication in individuals at high genetic risk of AD	2 – needs placebo-controlled prospective trials, about 67% risk reduction suggested	1 – high rates of adverse effects – anaemia, gastric irritation and bleeding
Hypertension	Antihypertensive medication and diet in people with high blood pressure, history of stroke or TIA	4 – vascular dementia but only modest reduction 3 – Alzheimer's disease	2 – most agents have the potential for adverse effects but other health benefits

cont.

Risk factor	Prevention strategy	Strength of evidence 0 = no evidence 1 = weak 2 = modest 3 = strong 4 = proven	Tolerability 0 = intolerable 1 = low 2 = moderate 3 = very tolerable
Smoking	Stop smoking	3 – vascular dementia 2 – Alzheimer's disease	3 – unlikely to harm and likely to have other health benefits
Cholesterol	Statins, diet in those with high cholesterol	2 – needs placebo-controlled prospective trials for AD and vascular dementia	2 – most agents have the potential for adverse effects but other health benefits
Cerebral blood flow – general – atherosclerosis	Ginkgo biloba Antiplatelet medication (aspirin)	0 – major controlled trials ineffective in preventing dementia 1 – vascular dementia 0 – Alzheimer's disease	2 – usually well tolerated but may cause bleeding 1 – high rates of adverse effects – anaemia, gastric irritation and bleeding
Diabetes mellitus	Diet, weight loss, better control of diabetes	2 – vascular dementia and Alzheimer's disease	3 – unlikely to harm and likely to have other health benefits

Risk factor	Prevention strategy	Strength of evidence 0 = no evidence 1 = weak 2 = modest 3 = strong 4 = proven	Tolerability 0 = intolerable 1 = low 2 = moderate 3 = very tolerable
Head injuries	Approved helmets for those at risk – boxers, bike riders	2 – the potential to reduce dementia is modest	2 – some find them too restrictive to wear
Delirium	Multifaceted delirium prevention programmes for hospitalised older people	1 – unclear whether it causes dementia or uncovers pre-clinical dementia	3 – unlikely to harm and likely to have other health benefits
General anaesthetics	Use local anaesthetics wherever feasible	1 – unclear whether it causes dementia or uncovers pre-symptomatic dementia	1 – may cause some discomfort for individuals
Electromagnetic radiation	Better shielding of electric motors in workplaces	1 – more studies required	2 – unlikely to harm but may have economic effects
Fumigants/ defoliants/ pesticides	Better protective clothing for workers at risk	1 – more studies required	2 – unlikely to harm but may have economic effects

cont.

Strength of evidence
0 = no evidence
1 = weak
2 = modest
3 = strong
4 = proven

Tolerability
0 = intolerable
1 = low
2 = moderate
3 = very tolerable

Risk factor	Prevention strategy	Strength of evidence	Tolerability
2. Indicated prevention – individuals with early symptoms or signs of dementia			
Mild cognitive impairment	Cognitive-enhancing drugs	1 – strong evidence of risk but no evidence of benefit from strategy	2 – most agents have the potential for adverse effects in 20–30%
Depression	Prevention of depression e.g. through better vascular health and improved coping skills	1 – modest evidence of risk but no evidence of benefit from strategy	3 – unlikely to harm and likely to have other health benefits
Post-traumatic stress disorder	Early intervention after trauma	1 – modest evidence of risk but no evidence of benefit from strategy	2 – disputed benefits in preventing PTSD

Key: AD = Alzheimer's disease

CHAPTER 4

The Symptoms and Course of Dementia

In most circumstances, dementia is a progressive condition that results in an evolving pattern of symptoms, behaviours, functional impairments and disabilities. The nature of an individual's presenting symptoms and the pattern of evolution will provide clues to the underlying type of dementia. For example, Alzheimer's disease tends to develop almost imperceptibly and progress gradually over a course that may run, on average, for 6 to 12 years. Vascular dementia has a more varied presentation and course, but a common variant is of relatively sudden onset followed by a stepwise decline over a somewhat shorter time span than seen in Alzheimer's disease. There are also many different symptoms of dementia as seen in Box 4.1.

Box 4.1 Symptoms of dementia

Memory impairment

Disorientation and confusion

Impaired language skills

Behavioural changes

Psychological symptoms, e.g. depression, anxiety and psychosis

Impaired judgement, insight and decision-making

Intellectual decline

Impaired functional capacity

Impaired social function

Because for most persons dementia is a chronic disorder, it is useful to view the course of dementia in stages according to the severity of the disease process. Note that these stages should be viewed only as a rough guide, since they are mainly based upon the course of Alzheimer's disease, not the other types of dementia. Further, some people may have some features from one stage and other features from an earlier or later stage. Specific cognitive and behavioural symptoms occur as damage afflicts various brain areas, as noted in Table 4.1.[1, 2]

Table 4.1 Brain areas, behaviour and cognition

Brain area	Dementia symptoms
Temporal lobe (includes the hippocampus)	Severe short-term memory impairment – difficulty with acquisition of new information for verbal and non-verbal material; word-finding difficulties; inability to recognise familiar faces; difficulty in naming objects in categories e.g. fruit, animals; aggressive behaviour; psychosis; depression
Frontal lobe	Difficulties in speech – expressive aphasia that lacks fluency and is impoverished; impaired organisation, planning, decision-making and judgement (executive skills); social behaviour impaired, e.g. sexual, manners, ability to empathise; social withdrawal, depression and apathy; short-term memory impairment – mainly in retrieving information often with confabulation (filling in gaps with false information); psychosis
Parietal lobe	Fluent speech but with difficulties in both comprehension and expression, use of paraphasias (substituting incorrect word e.g. 'spoon' instead of 'knife'); difficulties in processing of auditory information, e.g. unable to recognise familiar music, voices; lack of awareness of cognitive deficits; visuospatial impairments including neglect of parts of visual fields; difficulties in tactile recognition of familiar objects; difficulties with calculations
Subcortical structures – basal ganglia, thalamus, brainstem	Difficulties in speech; apathy; memory impairment with confabulation; poor attention and concentration; sleep/wake cycle changes; appetite changes; impaired organisation, planning, decision-making and judgement (executive skills)
Occipital lobe	Not often involved in dementia but can affect visual orientation and visual recognition of objects

Symptoms tend to develop at different times over the course of the dementia due to the order in which various parts of the brain become affected by the disease process. One particularly important brain area is the hippocampus in the temporal lobe, which is critical for short-term memory function and is damaged early in the course of Alzheimer's disease. The variability between individuals in the degree of damage that occurs in different parts of the brain over the course of dementia contributes to the broad spectrum of clinical patterns of disease. It is also important to understand that areas of the brain do not function independently but interact in a complex system with damage in one part of the brain being compensated for in another. Thus some symptoms might occur with damage in several different brain areas.

Pre-dementia – mild cognitive impairment

As with most illnesses, there is no set pattern of early symptoms. Presentations can be quite varied and are often recognised retrospectively. Furthermore, early symptoms may be subtle and attributable to many causes, a problem accentuated by dementia's relatively slow progression. Currently, we have limited knowledge of these earliest symptoms of dementia, and of how they might be distinguished from normal ageing and other mental conditions, although it does seem that when recall of new material is poor and not improved by cues, there is a higher risk of Alzheimer's disease. As pre-dementia merges almost imperceptibly with early dementia, the symptoms are discussed in more detail in the next section.

Mild or early-stage dementia

People with early dementia are able to function independently in most aspects of their life. Long-acquired social skills can compensate for their impairments, so it is not surprising to find that many acquaintances are unaware there is any problem at all. In fact, a mistake that some family members make after a dementia diagnosis has been made is to 'cotton wool' the person with dementia and not allow them to lead as normal a life as possible.

Short-term memory impairment is usually the most prominent early symptom of Alzheimer-type dementia. Such impairment results in the afflicted person having difficulty in remembering recent events – where they put the keys an hour ago, what their daughter told them on the phone last night, what they did last weekend. Contrary to popular belief, most

people are aware of deterioration in their memory. The majority, however, lack insight about the extent of their deficits and tend to deny that it is really impacting on their lives. When interviewed with family members present, upraised family eyebrows often accompany denial of the severity of the problem. More remote memories from childhood, adolescence and early adulthood are relatively unaffected in the early stage of dementia, yet in most cases, probing questions will reveal mild deficits, such as making minor mistakes in the chronology of their life history. Some people are very insightful about their memory loss and are acutely aware that it is abnormal. In my observation, the increased community awareness of dementia and Alzheimer's disease has resulted in more people presenting for assessment with a subjective awareness of their memory deficits.

> *For several years, Mary's family had noticed that she was becoming more forgetful. She frequently lost her keys and on two occasions had to have her front door locks changed. She seemed to forget telephone conversations that she had with her daughter, Alice. In one instance this resulted in Alice waiting for her mother at the shopping centre for over an hour, to have Mary say later that Alice must have been mistaken, as she hadn't been told about the arrangement. Despite these occurrences, Mary seemed to be coping quite well by herself, albeit more slowly and with fewer social outings. Alice wasn't too concerned – after all, her mother was 81 and 'Don't we all lose our memory as we get older?' It was only when Mary started to accuse her daughter of stealing her belongings when she visited her that Alice wondered whether there was something more seriously wrong. It was at this point that Alice decided to approach her mother's doctor about her concerns.*

This is a typical case history in which there has been a presumption that persistent memory impairment is due to age-related changes. It is only when other behavioural changes are superimposed upon the memory disturbance that action is taken. It is to be hoped that improved community awareness about dementia will result in more people being referred for assessment as soon as memory changes are detected. Short-term memory can be affected by numerous conditions, some of which include depression, stress, hearing loss, infections, medications, tumours, cerebrovascular disease and inflammatory disorders, in addition to age-related changes to memory function. Distinguishing normal ageing from the effects of such conditions and from dementia is one of the aims of dementia assessment.

Word-finding difficulties (aphasias) are also common, particularly with types of dementia that mainly involve the parietal and temporal cortical areas of the brain, for example Alzheimer's disease and frontotemporal dementia. Aphasia results in difficulties in finding the correct word for an object or the name of a familiar person. It can be manifested in several ways – the person might say 'the thing that holds the watch on the wrist' instead of 'watch band', or they will simply stop mid-sentence and express frustration with their efforts to find the right word. Others will report that they can no longer reliably remember the names of friends and acquaintances. There is also evidence that for some years before Alzheimer's disease becomes apparent, the person with dementia may have difficulties in understanding speech when there is a lot of background noise or competing signals. For people who speak English as a second language, aphasia may show itself in other ways.

> Angelo migrated to Australia from southern Italy in the 1950s to work on the Snowy Mountains Hydro-electric Scheme. He had limited education in Italy and spoke no English when he arrived but after a couple of years he spoke enough to get by, and by the 1960s spoke fluently albeit with a thick Italian accent. At the age of 73, Angelo's short-term memory began to decline. To the consternation of his family, he also started to have trouble finding the correct English word when he spoke and would substitute an Italian word instead. Within a few years, Angelo was speaking a hybrid of English and Italian and seemed to understand conversations in Italian best. This created problems for his grandchildren, who did not speak Italian.

There is a general rule with dementia – 'last in, first out'. Languages and other skills acquired later in life are usually the first skills lost as the dementia progresses. Thus people from a non-English speaking background characteristically lose their English language skills before their native tongue is affected.

Personality and behavioural changes are initially very subtle and usually attributed by family members and friends to age, stress, depression and sundry other causes. Dementias that involve the frontal lobe of the brain – frontotemporal dementia, vascular dementia and sometimes Alzheimer's disease – are particularly prone to this presentation. The slightly reserved, considerate person may start telling risqué jokes and committing repeated faux pas. The responsible, conservative investor may gradually take increased risks on the stock market. The placid, agreeable husband may become irritable, argumentative and temperamental. An outgoing, sociable wife may lose interest in going out with her friends and become generally

apathetic in her outlook. The meticulously groomed woman may start going out with poorly applied cosmetics and stained clothing.

In many cases, rather than a change to the opposite, there is an exacerbation of pre-morbid personality traits. The temperamental, verbally abusive husband turns to physical violence. The quiet, shy person becomes withdrawn and subdued. The easily worried, emotional person becomes persistently anxious, clingy and insecure. The suspicious, guarded loner becomes overtly paranoid.

Such personality and behavioural changes will clearly have an impact upon the person's lifestyle, resulting in family tensions and disruption of long-standing friendships. Sometimes the family doctor is consulted, though often nothing specific can be found. It is usually when other symptoms occur and the diagnosis of dementia is made that the family may become aware that the changed personality and behaviour is part of the dementia. At times irreparable damage may be done to relationships before the cause becomes clear. This is one situation where an early assessment by a psychiatrist or neurologist to clarify the cause of the changes may possibly limit the damage to family and social relationships.

Depression may be an early feature of dementia. Sometimes the clinical depression shows no hint of dementia and responds to antidepressant therapy, the other symptoms of dementia emerging months or years later. At other times, repeated efforts to treat what appear to be depressive symptoms are unsuccessful, or are only partially effective. In these situations, apathy due to frontal lobe impairment often obscures the dementia diagnosis. In a third situation there is a mix of depressive symptoms and memory changes, and it may be unclear for some time whether the memory problems are due to the depression or to early dementia.[3] The circumstance where depression is mistaken for dementia (pseudodementia) is discussed in Chapter 6.

At 68, Mark seemed to have reached a dead end. He had retired from the public service when he was 63 and, together with his wife Annette, he initially led a very active lifestyle that encompassed overseas travel, voluntary work and plenty of exercise. He was a passionate golfer, playing with his wife and friends several times a week. But over the last two years, he gradually gave up all of these pursuits, preferring instead to sit around at home all day. No matter how hard Annette and his friends tried to encourage him, he remained uninterested. He just couldn't understand their concerns. He seemed happy but had lost all motivation. There were no marital problems, though Annette was starting to lose her patience with him. His doctor had

prescribed several courses of antidepressant medication with no effect. At this stage, he was referred for assessment by an old age psychiatrist.

It is not surprising that this type of history would suggest depression as a possible cause of Mark's symptoms. Indeed, I would be concerned if he hadn't been treated with reasonable trials of antidepressant therapy. In the early stages, damage to the frontal lobes of the brain can be very difficult to distinguish from depression and investigations may be inconclusive. This is often very frustrating for family caregivers, who do not know where they stand.

Acute confusional episodes include symptoms of disorientation, perplexity, agitation, visual hallucinations and delusions (irrational false beliefs). Typically they are transient, usually lasting minutes to hours though sometimes for a few days. In early dementia, these episodes tend to occur mainly in vascular dementia, dementia with Lewy bodies and dementia associated with Parkinson's disease.

Such episodes are possibly most commonly associated with the transient confusion and hallucinations that may occur when waking from a dream at night. This is an extension of the normal phenomenon of 'hypnopompic hallucination' that many of us have experienced on awakening – a state in which it may take seconds to minutes to realise that we are still dreaming. The difference is that the acute confusional episode usually lasts longer and the person experiencing it may take some time to be reassured, as they tend to have poor insight into what has happened. Also, such episodes tend to start happening repeatedly.

Another common scenario is that in which a person becomes temporarily lost and disoriented when in a familiar locale, for example when driving or shopping. Sometimes this may overlap with short-term memory lapses when a car is left in a shopping centre car park and cannot be found. Again, with assistance from another person or after a short period of reflection, the confusion often settles.

Post-operative confusion after routine surgery may also be the first sign of early dementia. Frequently there is an underlying medical reason for the confusion, for example, infection or blood loss, but the mere fact that confusion has occurred at all is often a warning sign. Usually the confusion settles within days with appropriate treatment but sometimes it is clear to the family that full recovery hasn't occurred. In many cases, the confusion has merely added to subtle signs of memory or personality change which had been noticed before the surgery. Occasionally there

are no pre-operative symptoms, and the possibility that there has been an adverse intra-operative event must be considered.

> At 85, Daisy had become rather frail. Her bones were weakened by osteoporosis and arthritis and her mobility was poor. She also had high blood pressure, diabetes and asthma, and suffered from constipation, which led to her being prescribed ten different medications a day by a variety of medical specialists and her local doctor. Despite these problems, her family felt she was 'reasonably alert' and only occasionally forgetful. It came as no surprise, however, when she fell and fractured her hip. Twenty-four hours after surgery, her son was called from the hospital to be informed that Daisy was severely confused, agitated and calling out. This improved over the next fortnight but she remained more forgetful, less alert and indecisive. Her family were convinced that something must have happened during the operation.

Another occasional situation where acute confusional states may herald the appearance of dementia is illustrated by the following case.

> David and Joan were travelling through Europe on a coach tour. One night at 3am an agitated Joan rudely woke David. She told him that something strange had happened to their home – the bathroom had been moved. Initially David had enormous difficulty convincing her that they were in a hotel room in Europe. She seemed to really believe that she was at home in New York but eventually settled with reassurance. David didn't think much more about it as the next day Joan was back to her normal self. When informed about what had happened, she could barely recall it so they both just shrugged it off as a bad dream. A few nights later, in a different hotel, Joan again woke David in the middle of the night with the same concern. This time she wasn't easily reassured and also expressed the belief that possibly the neighbours were responsible and were trying to trick her. After an hour, David became so concerned that he called for the hotel doctor, who arranged for a hospital assessment. Joan's confusion settled within hours and no significant acute medical problems were detected. Joan was advised to have a more detailed examination when she returned to the US.

As more retirees travel, this type of scenario is occurring more frequently. Of course, disorientation and confusion in unfamiliar surroundings are a common problem that can spoil holidays for both people with dementia and their caregivers. Taking precautions when travelling, such as always having a familiar caregiver present, keeping the travel time as short as possible, taking familiar bedside objects to put into the new bedroom,

having plenty of rest periods, maintaining hydration, exercise and avoiding alcohol can all help to minimise problems.

Moderate or middle-stage dementia

Probably the major feature that distinguishes moderate dementia from mild dementia is the clear need for the person with dementia to be provided with some level of assistance to maintain their function in the community to as near as possible to the level they enjoyed before the onset of the dementia.

Memory and orientation

At the moderate stage of dementia, memory function is severely affected. Memories of recent events are very poorly retained, though verbal and visual reminders or cues may elicit some recall in some people. Mentioning a friend's name might be a reminder of a visit to their home. Showing a picture of a relative might remind them of a birthday. If the event that has just happened has great emotional significance to the person, recall is likely to be better. For example, the death of a spouse in the previous week is likely to be remembered to some degree, while a routine bus trip would not. This was demonstrated graphically in Japan some years ago after a major earthquake. Many nursing home residents with dementia could remember the earthquake, but not recent, mundane, day-to-day events.

Remote memories are also more overtly affected. While the person with dementia will still dwell in the past, their reminiscences are repetitive and lacking in detail. The chronological sequence of past events is now certainly disrupted. Their wedding day may occur before they were born, the birthdays of children are entangled and ages are mere estimates. Even knowledge of where their wedding occurred, their place of employment and details of important world events such as World War II are usually faulty.

Disorientation in time is a constant. There is little chance of knowing the day, date or month of the year, though they may know the year. The usual response is along the lines that 'all days seem the same' or 'it really doesn't matter what day it is'. Orientation in place will depend on where they are. Usually disoriented in unfamiliar surroundings, in their own home they will, as a rule, know where they are. Trips to new or only vaguely familiar places may provoke anxiety and confusion. However, repeat visits to a new place that is perceived as being friendly and relaxing, such as a dementia day care centre, will usually quell anxiety; and the person with

dementia may attain a degree of orientation to it. There are exceptions to this, as noted in the following scenario.

> Raymond had been diagnosed with Alzheimer's disease four years ago and was cared for by Jennifer, his wife. She had been able to look after him without too much concern until one day he demanded to be taken home – when he was sitting in his lounge room. Taken aback, Jennifer initially didn't know what to say but after reassuring him and showing him around the house, he settled down. Wisely, Jennifer had Raymond checked by their local doctor, who could find no evidence of any acute medical problem and advised her that it was likely to be part of the process of the dementia. These episodes started to happen on a regular basis and it became apparent that Raymond believed that he still lived in the home they used to occupy in a different suburb in the early years of their marriage. On one occasion he became so insistent that Jennifer even took him to the site of their long-demolished first home to convince him he was mistaken. Eventually she discovered that the only way to mollify Raymond was to take him out in the car, drive him around the block and pretend that they had arrived at their home.

This type of strategy doesn't work for everyone but is well worth trying. It is a good example of 'going with the flow' rather than trying to convince the person with dementia that they are mistaken.

Acute confusional episodes where there may be marked disorientation associated with behavioural changes, hallucinations and paranoia developing over hours to days, are now likely to occur when there is an infection or other acute medical condition.

Language and calculation

Naming difficulties are more noticeable in everyday speech. Names of familiar people and of common objects are regularly stumbled over. Less obvious to the casual listener but quite apparent to family and friends is the growing impoverishment of speech. The content has less detail, fewer spontaneous comments are made and much of what is said is repetitive. Indeed, repetitive utterances can cause enormous distress to caregivers, particularly when they take the form of a question. Despite the caregiver giving an answer, the same question may be asked minutes later…and again and again and again. This is called 'speech perseveration'. Another example is the same response being given repeatedly to different questions. Multilingual persons often use several languages simultaneously and are largely unaware they are doing so. The most recently acquired languages continue to erode the most quickly.

Comprehension is also more severely affected. What caregivers may interpret as poor memory may in fact be poor comprehension of what has been said. Complex commands may be misunderstood, sometimes to the extent that a hearing deficit is suspected and a hearing aid considered. In similar vein, comprehension of written material is also poor. This, in combination with diminished concentration, memory and motivation, usually results in a marked reduction of time spent in reading. Caregivers will note that the same page in the book has been 'read' for days or weeks.

Simple calculations may no longer be reliably completed, particularly without pen and paper. This is most noticeable when shopping, where the person with dementia often relies completely on the honesty of the shop assistant to give the correct change. Even if given their date of birth and the current date, it is also unlikely that they will be able to calculate their age.

Executive and intellectual function

Executive function, largely a function of the frontal lobes of the brain, can be equated with managerial skills. A decline in intellectual skills is noted by an inability to solve day-to-day problems, learn new skills (for example, how to operate a new appliance) or appreciate abstract aspects of relationships. Organisational and planning abilities become progressively impaired. The person with dementia may repeatedly say they are going to do something but never get around to doing it. In this way, hobbies and other life-long interests are progressively abandoned. Skills acquired earliest are usually retained longer – 'first in, last out'. Judgement and insight about their own capacity may be poor, with a failure to recognise their own limitations. This may also extend to judgements about others, as can be seen in the following case.

> Julie had always been friendly and enjoyed company. Despite her dementia, she still lived alone with support from family and neighbours. When a young man with a hard luck story knocked on the door and offered to do some odd jobs for her, she felt obliged to help out. She paid him $30 to do $10 worth of shopping. Unsurprisingly, he returned regularly, usually after pension day, and was paid well each time for very small jobs. She felt unable to refuse despite having a nagging feeling that she should. A pensioner, she had always been careful with her finances. Her family started to become concerned when Julie kept asking to borrow money. They noted that several large sums of money had been withdrawn from her bank accounts shortly after pension day. Julie told them a vague story of a destitute young man who had been helping her.

I regularly assess people with dementia in their homes and am constantly amazed about how trusting most people are with strangers. While this makes my job easier, it is also apparent how vulnerable many people with dementia are to fraud.

Self-care and functional capacity

It is during this stage that capacity to self-care declines; it is particularly noticeable in people who live alone. Personal hygiene, dressing, cooking, shopping, financial management and social skills become impaired. Usually the person with dementia doesn't recognise the need for assistance, due to their impaired judgement and insight, and may only grudgingly accept help. Many persons with moderate dementia are living alone in the community with minimal or no assistance. Almost inevitably, this is achieved by accepting a reduction in their standard of living, for example, by living in dirty conditions, by wearing soiled clothing, by eating little food of dubious freshness, by socialising minimally or by having financial problems through forgetting to pay bills.

Mavis had lived alone since her husband died ten years earlier. She had always looked after herself without needing to call on her daughter Jane, who lived interstate, though she maintained regular phone contact and visited each year. For some years Mavis had been getting more forgetful. She and Jane put it down to age now that Mavis had reached 78. During her previous visit, Jane had noticed that the usually impeccably clean home was rather untidy (as was Mavis herself), that the customarily well-stocked refrigerator contained plenty of milk (much of it out of date) and only a few other odds and ends, and that several unopened power and water bills lay on the kitchen table. Mavis had explained this by saying she had been 'sick with a virus' and was just about to do it all. After Jane had helped her mother clean the house, pay the bills and restock the fridge, she suggested that maybe it was time that she accepted some regular help with the shopping and housework. It was like a red rag to a bull. Mavis angrily told her daughter that she didn't need any help and that if this was 'the sort of way that you are going to treat me' then she would be better off not visiting. She quickly calmed down, however, and by the time Jane returned home all was forgiven. Over the next six months, Jane phoned at least weekly and often every few days as she became increasingly concerned about the extent of her mother's forgetfulness and poor self-care. She quickly gained the impression that unless she reminded Mavis to shop and pay bills, little would be done. An earlier than usual visit was arranged, not that Mavis noticed. Jane was shocked to see how messy her

mother's home had become and the apparent lack of concern. Mavis was wearing a heavily soiled dress and smelt as if she hadn't bathed for weeks. Despite Jane's phone calls, the fridge was again bare and unopened bills lay on the table. As before, Mavis claimed she had just had a 'virus' but otherwise she felt okay and didn't need any help.

This is a common type of scenario, leading family members to difficult choices about when and how to insist that some type of community service be introduced to help the person with dementia cope at home. It frequently leads to referrals to aged care services, geriatricians and old age psychiatrists which ensures that the person with dementia is thoroughly assessed, that an accurate diagnosis is obtained and the prognosis is outlined.

For some caregivers, it comes as a surprise to be told that the changes in self-care and function are due to dementia, not age. When they know what the future is likely to hold, however, both the person with dementia and caregiver are in a better position to plan even at this relatively late stage of the disease.

When the person with dementia is living with a caregiver, usually a spouse, many self-care and functional capacity issues are effectively concealed to the outside world as the caregiver gradually takes on more and more tasks. Sometimes the transfer of responsibilities is achieved almost imperceptibly over some years, and without any dramas. For example, the person with dementia may be gently reminded to have a shower, clean clothes will appear after the shower and the dirty ones removed surreptitiously, and dressing will be monitored to ensure the clothes are put on correctly. Often the degree of dependence only comes to light in a crisis, for example, when the caregiver becomes acutely unwell, and it comes as a great surprise to friends and other family members that the person with dementia is so incapacitated.

Of course, for the person with dementia to transition from independence to partial dependence doesn't always go smoothly and can become the source of much conflict with the caregiver. Issues that often lead to disputes include financial management, driving, personal hygiene and social activities. These are discussed in more detail in later chapters.

Behavioural changes

It is in this stage of dementia that behavioural changes become more marked, occurring to a significant degree in approximately 50 per cent of cases. There is evidence that there are neurobiological alterations in the

brain that contribute to the behavioural changes.[4] The neurotransmitters serotonin, dopamine and noradrenaline have been associated with behaviour changes that include aggression, agitation and psychosis. In general, increasing severity of neuropathology in Alzheimer's disease is associated with increased risk of psychosis. Reduced function in the frontal lobes, as determined by low perfusion on neuroimaging, has been associated with apathy, depression and psychosis, while reduced function in the temporal lobes has been associated with psychosis, depression and aggression.[5]

Studies have demonstrated that challenging behaviours and associated psychological symptoms are strongly associated with caregiver stress and placement of the person with dementia into residential care.[6] Not all changes of behaviour are a problem. Often an explanation to the caregiver that the behaviour change is part of the dementia allows the caregiver to tolerate it. At other times the behaviour itself is not abnormal, it is just occurring in the wrong place or at the wrong time. Other behaviours can be more of a challenge.

ACTIVITY DISTURBANCES

Wandering occurs in 30 to 40 per cent of cases and may become a serious concern.[7] 'Wandering' is an all-encompassing term covering a broad range of behaviours that involve a change in the physical activity of the person with dementia and/or their ability to find their way back home. In moderate dementia, wandering behaviours mainly involve an element of disorientation – the person with dementia becomes lost and attempts unsuccessfully to find their way home. Sometimes they use common sense and get a cab or ask for help; more frequently a Good Samaritan notices their confusion and provides assistance. Often this occurs after a considerable period of walking. At other times, the desire to walk simply increases without necessarily involving any disorientation. Long daily walks around the neighbourhood occur, often to the concern of family members, who fear the person with dementia will either get lost or accidentally walk in front of a car. Sometimes the walking is aimless and associated with general restlessness; at other times there is a particular purpose. One example of purposeful wandering can occur in the situation described in the previous vignette where Raymond would start wandering from his current home in a search for his previous home.

Underactivity can also occur and is usually associated with general apathy and amotivation. Some people with dementia take to their bed for

no apparent reason and appear happy to have caregivers provide for their every need. This can be very frustrating for the caregiver.

AGGRESSIVE BEHAVIOUR

Aggressive behaviour is one of the more difficult behaviours for caregivers to cope with, but many bear with it for a considerable time before requesting help. It can occur in a number of circumstances. In some cases, the aggression appears to be associated with hallucinations and paranoid delusions that seem to be the spur for a range of behaviour from verbal abuse and irritability to actual violence. Occasionally serious assaults may ensue. Treatment of the psychosis reduces the risk of dangerousness. Aggressive behaviour also can occur without psychotic symptoms through a coarsening of the pre-morbid personality, low frustration tolerance, depression or disinhibition. Often aggression only occurs when assistance is required with personal care and in this circumstance it could be interpreted as a reaction to a perceived threat. The person with dementia may simply be uncooperative; sometimes actual physical aggression occurs.

> Tamara had always regarded her husband, Rupert, as a gentleman. Throughout their marriage he had been courteous, caring and supportive to her and their children. As his Alzheimer-type dementia unfolded, some early signs of personality change became quite pronounced. Four years after diagnosis, Rupert was now easily irritated and would swear at Tamara when frustrated, using four-letter words she had never heard from him before. Sometimes he would push her, which on several occasions resulted in bruises. This marked change in Rupert's personality and behaviour was extremely distressing for Tamara, but she felt that to tell her children, friends or doctor about what was happening would be a betrayal of her husband. So she kept it to herself, largely by severely limiting her social contacts and giving a range of increasingly improbable excuses for her bruises to her children and friends. Eventually, after a particularly distressing incident, she realised that she needed help and consulted her doctor.

This is not an unusual story. Wives in particular often tolerate quite disturbed behaviour for a long time before seeking help. Embarrassment, obligation and sometimes fear prevent many from getting assistance. Of course, other caregivers do not tolerate even relatively minor behavioural changes and seek help at an early stage.

SLEEP DISTURBANCE

One of the effects of neuropathological changes in the brainstem is a disruption of the sleep–wake cycle. At times the sleep disturbance can

resemble sleep apnea. Sleep patterns progressively deteriorate as the dementia worsens, more so in people who have previously been poor sleepers. Sleep periods become shorter, shallower and more frequent, so it becomes common to have naps during the day and periods of wakefulness at night. At its extreme, day–night reversal of sleep patterns can occur. Caregivers often face a similar situation to mothers of restless babies, becoming sleep deprived themselves with consequent irritability, poor concentration and symptoms of depression.

DISINHIBITED BEHAVIOUR

Disinhibited behaviours occur where there has been an impairment of the psychological processes that restrain the expression of instinctual drives. In people with dementia this usually occurs due to frontal lobe damage. There are certain behaviours that we learn very early are socially inappropriate – picking our noses in public, walking down the street without clothes, touching another person without consent, telling complete strangers intimate personal details, and so on. When these behaviours occur as a result of dementia, family and friends are often very distressed. Disinhibited sexual behaviours can be particularly upsetting. Most persons with moderate dementia do not engage in regular sexual activity, but occasionally libido appears to increase and their partner may be repeatedly propositioned every day. Occasionally sexual molestation of caregivers may occur, particularly in residential care. Often this takes the form of fondling breasts and bottoms. In some cases the behaviour may represent an inappropriate way of trying to express intimacy needs.

Psychological symptoms

Often linked with behavioural changes, it is useful to conceptualise them separately as these symptoms are often quite distressing to the person with dementia whereas behavioural changes usually only bother other people. It is not surprising that moderate dementia should cause a wide range of psychological symptoms, for it is during this stage that the impact of declining cognition and function really becomes noticeable. Even though their impaired insight may serve to limit the impact, most people with dementia will, if given the opportunity, express their difficulties in understanding their changing world in a variety of ways.

MISINTERPRETATIONS, ILLUSIONS AND PSYCHOSIS

Misinterpretations and illusions become prevalent and take many forms. Relatives are accused of stealing misplaced objects, familiar people are

misidentified, normal neighbourhood noise is misconstrued as machinery, and friends are accused of talking about them behind their back. This especially occurs at night, when sensory stimuli are fewer, and in unfamiliar surroundings. Another important factor may be the presence of a visual agnosia due to the dementia, which results in the person being unable to recognise common objects despite otherwise normal eyesight. Sometimes a simple demonstration of where lost objects are located, or an explanation of the misinterpreted event, allied with reassurance, will result in the person's acceptance of being mistaken – although this problem is likely to recur.

At other times no amount of explanation or reassurance will alter their beliefs. There is usually a sense of persecution and suspicion. In these circumstances, the beliefs have become delusional and the person with dementia is regarded as having a psychosis. One particularly distressing type of delusion is illustrated in the next case.

> Joseph and Eva had been married for 53 years. They had a devoted relationship in which neither had contemplated life without the other. They met in a refugee camp after World War II, having both narrowly escaped death in the Holocaust. After marrying, they resettled in Australia and decided that they were not prepared to have children. Throughout their marriage they kept to themselves and had few friends. At the age of 82, Joseph had a mild stroke in which he became briefly confused and unsteady on his feet. Subsequently, Eva noticed that he started to have memory lapses, which worsened six months later after another mild stroke. Of greater concern, he became irritable and intermittently started to accuse Eva of having an affair with a neighbour. Her reassurances only served to anger him. She felt devastated by the turn of events. Fortunately her doctor was very supportive and managed to convince Joseph to take an antipsychotic drug, and after a few weeks his delusions lessened and he stopped persecuting Eva.

This type of delusion is known as 'morbid jealousy'. Unfortunately there is a high risk of physical assaults in these situations, so control of the delusions with medication is often crucial. Morbid jealousy can occur in many situations apart from dementia and is not always due to a psychosis. Some people are just inherently jealous and while they may not actually believe their partner is unfaithful, they constantly query their fidelity and may even search for signs that an affair has occurred.

Visual and auditory hallucinations may also occur but usually in association with delusions. People and animals may be seen, neighbours' conversations may be overheard from quite a distance, strange machinery

noises perceived. It is sometimes difficult to know whether there is any factual basis to the experience. For example, it is not uncommon for the person who believes that he can overhear his neighbours to be living in an apartment with thin walls through which noises are easily transmitted. Another issue is that hallucinations are much more likely to occur in people with hearing and visual deficits. Sometimes the 'noises' heard are really tinnitus, but this explanation is not often readily accepted; usually the person with dementia prefers a delusional interpretation, such as the neighbours using a new electronic gadget to keep him or her awake at night. Hallucinations are particularly common in dementia with Lewy bodies, which is described in Chapter 5.

DEPRESSION

Depressive symptoms occur in up to 50 per cent of moderate dementias. A far lower percentage experience actual clinical depression. Depression may occur as a psychological reaction to declining mental function, as an exaggeration of pre-morbid traits, or as an inherent part of the dementia due to changes in brain neurotransmitters. Depression may be difficult to diagnose in a person with dementia but should be suspected if they wish to die or have suicidal ideas, where there has been an otherwise unexplained sudden decline in function or change in behaviour (for example aggression or reduced appetite), or if the person is tearful for no apparent reason. As mentioned previously when describing symptoms of early dementia, distinguishing depression from frontal lobe apathy is also not easy.[8]

ANXIETY

Symptoms of anxiety are also common and often occur in association with depression. Anxiety symptoms are more likely to occur in a pre-morbidly anxious person. Intense fear of abandonment by the caregiver is an especially challenging situation in which the person with dementia won't let their spouse leave them for even a few minutes without becoming very agitated. This can lead to the caregiver feeling trapped. At times these fears can reach delusional intensity. When the anxious person with dementia lives alone, frequent phone calls to family and friends for reassurance are likely to occur. This may happen many times every day, to the intense frustration of the recipients. The anxiety often improves dramatically in company, indicating that the person with dementia may be lonely. This presents the obvious solution of living with others, either with family, friends or in a long-term care home, but there is generally a surprising degree of resistance to the suggestion.

Social function

In moderate dementia, independent social functioning has all but disappeared. While there may be a facade of normality, this is usually achieved by the efforts of an attentive caregiver or sensitive friends. Alone, the person with dementia is liable to make errors while shopping, travelling and banking, and they usually require the goodwill of service providers to get through. For many people, attempts to function independently in social situations are so anxiety-provoking that social activities are largely abandoned. For others, the loss of initiative and organisational skills largely prevent participation in social activities without someone else to arrange it. Friends who do not understand why they are no longer contacted by the person with dementia may incorrectly feel they are being snubbed and respond by ceasing to make contact themselves. This lack of social interaction may increase boredom and depression. It is often noted that when an organised social activity is regularly arranged, the person with dementia perks up.

Severe or late-stage dementia

By this stage of dementia, there is no semblance of independent function and the majority of persons with severe dementia are in residential care. Maintenance at home usually requires 24-hour care from family, friends and community support services. The level of care required is so intense over such a long time (usually at least a year or two) that, in the absence of an intercurrent illness, almost all persons with severe dementia eventually spend some time in residential care.

Memory and orientation

There is now very severe to profound memory impairment. There is virtually no recall of recent events and past memories are fragmentary and imprecise. Concentration is extremely poor and the person is very distractible during many tasks. In addition to being disoriented in time, there is now disorientation in place and, as the dementia worsens, disorientation to self, with the person being unable to cite their name. In married women this often announces itself initially when they start to respond with their maiden name.

Confusional episodes associated with any medical illness, medications, environmental changes, pain, constipation, and sundry other causes are the rule rather than the exception in severe dementia.

Language

Language skills are rapidly lost. Speech becomes increasingly impoverished, with the use of simple sentences or phrases, and very concrete interpretations of questions. There is little evidence of spontaneous conversation, with the majority of spontaneous utterances being a request for some form of help. Often the same words or phrases are repeated over and over again (perseveration). Many sufferers eventually completely lose their speech (become aphasic). Speech is replaced by various noises, somewhat like the range of sounds that pre-verbal infants use. In a similar fashion to infants, many of the sounds have meaning that perceptive caregivers are able to understand. And, like pre-verbal infants, loud repetitive utterances of late-stage dementia can be extremely stressful to caregivers.

> Anne had severe Alzheimer's disease and had been in the nursing home for a year. For the past six months her speech had been limited to a few words. Yet she would chatter continuously for hours at a time in a loud high-pitched voice. Most of the time she would repeat the same sounds over and over again – 'da-da-da-da-da', screeches, or sometimes, discernible words. Her noisiness was very disruptive to other residents and staff. Visitors complained, as did neighbours. It got to the stage that staff avoided her as they found her 'chattering' so stressful.

Comprehension appears to be more slowly eroded, though it is necessary to communicate using simple language slowly and often with associated gestures.

Executive and intellectual function

In severe dementia, there is very limited intellectual function. There is no semblance of capacity to organise and plan, the person with dementia being completely dependent on others. Decision-making is restricted to very simple choices and often impeded by poor judgement. Insight is minimal. There is often no recognition of the extent of incapacity and the person may become very angry and distressed about being unable to do things when they want to. This is one of the factors that contribute to some of the challenging behaviours in this stage of dementia that are discussed later. Yet, a partial ability to learn simple things may remain for a surprising amount of time, a capacity that allows caregivers to modulate some behaviour. Also, musical appreciation may be retained to the extent that the types of music that the person enjoyed in the past may still evoke enjoyment.

Self-care and functional capacity

During this stage of dementia, the person with dementia progresses from requiring assistance to toilet, bathe, eat and dress to being fully dependent on a caregiver to do these things for them. Self-care skills are rapidly lost without regular practice, so it is not unusual to see a marked decline in function after a prolonged illness such as pneumonia. Due to this tendency, caregivers are always encouraged to try to allow the person with dementia do as much for themselves as possible, though the dilemma may be that this takes an inordinate amount of time. Urinary and later faecal incontinence is universal, though this progresses in stages from occasional nocturnal incontinence, to incontinence that responds to regular toileting by others, to complete incontinence needing 24-hour continence pads. Swallowing problems are common, particularly in persons with vascular dementia, and may result in recurrent bouts of pneumonia caused by inhalation of food and stomach acid. Others simply stop eating, which raises the vexed question of tube feeding, discussed in Chapter 12. If the person with dementia doesn't die of an intercurrent illness (most frequently pneumonia, stroke or heart attack), eventually the ability to walk is lost and the person becomes initially chairbound and then bedbound.

Behavioural changes

Challenging behaviours reach a peak around the period of transition from moderate to severe dementia. Each of the behaviours described in moderate dementia continues to occur in severe dementia, though as functional impairment becomes more marked and physical function declines, they tend to diminish. It should also be remembered that these behaviours are not universal, although as dementia progresses, non-verbal means of communication increase. Some behaviours in severe dementia are mainly a form of communication but the challenge to caregivers (and part of the reason for the term 'challenging behaviour' rather than 'problem behaviour') is to determine their meaning.

ACTIVITY DISTURBANCES

While overactivity prompts most concern in severe dementia, activity levels generally reduce and many people become quite inert without prompting from caregivers. This underactivity can be a major problem, contributing to sleep disruption and boredom. General restlessness and aimless wandering are the predominant overactivity disturbances. One situation that causes a lot of concern is where a person who is unable to

walk safely without assistance insists on walking alone and repeatedly falls over. Physical restraints can be applied to stop the falls, but this is not an appropriate strategy and has the consequence of increasing their agitation and distress. Some who are bedbound will writhe around so forcefully that they throw themselves out of bed.

UNCOOPERATIVE BEHAVIOURS

Many challenging behaviours in severe dementia reflect a clash between a person with dementia lacking insight, who wants to do or not do something, and a caregiver who is either trying to prevent the person with dementia from endangering themselves or to assist them with a function. As the person with dementia's functional capacity diminishes, there are more and more occasions where hands-on physical assistance is required. Some people quite enjoy the help and are cooperative, others object to the loss of their autonomy, or feel embarrassed, or maybe simply don't like the particular person helping them or the way they are being helped. Sometimes even well-meaning staff can inadvertently be rough. Uncooperative behaviours can range from stubborn resistance to verbal and physical aggression. The following case is typical.

> Ricardo had severe vascular dementia and a hemiparesis from a recent stroke. He was completely dependent on the nursing home staff for all of his basic care. He was completely incontinent of urine and faeces but whenever the nursing staff tried to change him, he became very agitated, pushing them away and sometimes striking them. It reached a stage where the staff were reluctant to change him even though they knew this was untenable. Eventually, they found that he was more cooperative with male staff, and those who spoke his native Spanish.

Finding the right approach for the individual can be a challenge for both professional and informal caregivers. Sometimes the most unexpected things work. It is important that caregivers do not give up in their efforts to try different strategies, though each new strategy should be given a reasonable trial before being abandoned as unsuccessful.

EATING BEHAVIOUR

Eating behaviour changes in a variety of ways in moderate to severe dementia but 'refusal to eat' causes greatest concern, especially when it is associated with weight loss, which tends to happen with most persons with severe dementia anyway. 'Refusal to eat' encompasses a range of issues and in many cases is an inaccurate description of what is happening.

The coordination required to use knives and forks to feed declines due to the process of the dementia, and sometimes food left untouched simply reflects this loss of function. Most persons with severe dementia need to be fed, but some spit out food, push it away or won't open their mouths. As dementia becomes more severe, the ability to eat falls off. The masticatory process becomes uncoordinated, chewing may be ineffective, tongue movements may fail to prepare the food bolus to be swallowed, and the swallowing reflex may be incompetent. These are all good reasons for apparent food refusal. Other factors that may contribute to 'refusal to eat' include the quality of the food, ill-fitting or absent dentures, inability to see the food due to poor eyesight, and the lack of a social milieu that encourages eating. Many become concerned that food refusal may be due to the person with dementia 'giving up' in a depressed mood and occasionally this may be the case. In a nursing home study in Sydney that I undertook with Henry Brodaty and colleagues, we found that depression was not commonly associated with 'refusal to eat'.[9]

Other changes in eating behaviour, which may become apparent in earlier stages of dementia, include predilections for certain food such as sweets and chocolates, overeating, eating of inedible objects (pica) and an alteration in taste which may be related to a reduced sense of smell.

DISINHIBITED BEHAVIOUR
In severe dementia, the types of disinhibited behaviour that cause concern are varied. Intrusiveness and rummaging through other people's possessions are common. Usually the person with dementia has no idea that they are in someone else's room. Confrontations may occur, with violent outcomes. Vocally disruptive behaviour with repeated calling out for assistance or attention is a particularly distressing behaviour for staff and residents. Inappropriate sexual behaviours that tend to occur later in the dementia include exposure and masturbation in public.

Psychological symptoms
It is difficult to tell what the psychological processes of a person with severe dementia who is unable to speak coherently or write might be. Not least for this reason, studies of the symptoms of anxiety and depression show a decline in prevalence as dementia progresses. Interpretation of non-verbal communication would suggest that psychological reactions are still occurring but what they are is difficult to ascertain. Smiles, cries, frowns, winces all convey meaning that are almost certainly reflecting underlying emotional states, physical discomfort or pain.

Social function

While independent social function is no longer possible, social interactions remain important. In a non-threatening environment that caters for the limitations in their function, most persons with severe dementia thrive. Supervised dance, exercise, music, games and involvement with simple chores often provide surprising insights into quiescent abilities. Some people, of course, have never enjoyed social activities and won't change. Others are too distractible to stay for long.

Advanced dementia

Many people with dementia die before they reach the stage of advanced dementia, particularly if they have other significant health problems. By this stage the person with dementia is completely dependent on caregivers for all aspects of daily living and has almost certainly been in long-term residential care for some time. Language skills are lost and many are mute. Memory function is virtually impossible to test. Most are unable to stand or walk without assistance, many are unable to sit up properly. Due to their lack of activity, passive exercises are essential to prevent contractures of arms and legs, and routine pressure care is required to prevent the development of bedsores. Most long-term residential care homes have good pressure care routines but if residents with advanced dementia are transferred to hospital for any reason, there is a high risk that they will return with bedsores.[10] Acute hospitals seem to have difficulty in implementing pressure care effectively alongside all the other demands made on their staff. Feeding difficulties are almost universal and many are unable to swallow safely. This raises the issue of tube feeding, discussed in Chapter 12. Urinary and faecal incontinence is the rule. Most people with dementia die from infections (pneumonia, influenza), cardiac arrest or stroke.

Summary

Most types of dementia are gradually progressive as they course through mild, moderate, severe and advanced stages. This means that the symptoms of early dementia differ from those found at later stages. Apart from impairments in memory and orientation, the other symptom domains of dementia include language and calculation, executive and intellectual function, behaviour, psychological reactions, self-care and functional capacity, and social function.

CHAPTER 5

Types of Dementia

There are over one hundred established types of dementia, but most of them are extremely rare. In this chapter I will describe the four main types of dementia seen in clinical practice – Alzheimer's disease, vascular dementia, frontotemporal dementia and dementia with Lewy bodies – which account for 90 to 95 per cent of all cases – and a number of less common types, as listed in Table 5.1.[1, 2]

Table 5.1 Types of dementia

Common 90–95%

Alzheimer's disease 50–75%*
Vascular dementia 20–30%*
Dementia with Lewy bodies 5–20%*
Frontotemporal dementia 5–10%

* These categories overlap and include mixed Alzheimer's/vascular dementia up to 25%, mixed Alzheimer's/DLB up to 15%

Uncommon 5–10%

(a) Other neurodegenerative diseases

Parkinson's disease
Progressive supranuclear palsy
Cortico-basal degeneration
Creutzfeldt-Jakob disease
Huntington's disease
Familial British dementia

cont.

(b) Traumatic causes

Head injuries
Subdural haematoma

(c) Tumours

Brain tumours – primary and secondary

(d) Infections

HIV (AIDS dementia complex)
Neurosyphilis
Chronic meningitis
Viral encephalitis

(e) Toxic, metabolic and endocrine causes

Thyroid disorders
Vitamin B_{12} and folate deficiency
Metabolic disorders – chronic kidney and liver failure
Chronic drug intoxication e.g. long-term anti-epileptic medication
Alcohol-related dementia

(f) Other

Normal pressure hydrocephalus
Auto-immune disorders e.g. temporal arteritis
Anoxic brain damage e.g. after cardiac arrest
Multiple sclerosis

Previous chapters outlined the common risk factors for dementia and described the clinical features, albeit with a particular focus on Alzheimer's disease. Here my focus will be on what is understood about why these disorders occur and specific features that distinguish them from each other.

Apart from vascular dementia, most of the dementias are categorised as neurodegenerative disorders because essentially they involve the progressive degeneration and death of nerve cells. There is now mounting evidence for a common theme uniting these disorders. In a nutshell, neurodegenerative disorders are fundamentally caused by the abnormal accumulation of insoluble proteins in the brain. These proteins are toxic and exert a deleterious effect on selective nerve cells, impairing their function and eventually leading to cell death. The abnormal proteins

also affect synapses (spaces) between nerve cells, therefore the chemical information between cells might not be transmitted properly and nerve circuits might be interrupted.[3]

This is a fast-moving area with new discoveries happening almost every week. I concentrate on what seems to be reasonably well accepted by the scientific community rather than what is speculative.

Alzheimer's disease

Alzheimer's disease is the most common type of dementia, accounting for about 50 to 75 per cent of cases, although some of these cases are in combination with vascular dementia and/or dementia with Lewy bodies. It is named after the German neurologist Alois Alzheimer who first described the neuropathology (brain pathology) in a famous lecture in 1906. The patient was a woman in her 50s, Auguste Deter, who experienced symptoms of hallucinations, disorientation and memory loss that progressed over some years until her death at the age of 55 years. Alzheimer identified the two major abnormalities in the brain that characterise the disease – senile plaques and neurofibrillary tangles in the cortex of the brain.[4] His senior colleague, Emil Kraepelin, one of the founding figures of modern psychiatry, named the disease after Alzheimer.

For the next 60 or 70 years, Alzheimer's disease was considered to be a rare condition that caused pre-senile dementia in people under the age of 65 years. Senile dementia, which developed in late life, was regarded as a separate disorder. It was considered either as a normal part of the ageing process (senescence) or as due to arteriosclerotic changes (hardening of the arteries) in cerebral blood vessels.[5] However, research in Newcastle-upon-Tyne in the UK, published in the late 1960s and early 1970s, and from the US in the early 1970s demonstrated that senile dementia and Alzheimer's disease were the same condition.[6, 7, 8] This has led to the explosion of research over the last 40 years.

As described in detail in Chapter 4, Alzheimer's disease is a gradually progressive disorder that has a course of 6 to 12 years, though there have been people who have died within 12 months and others who have survived for more than 20 years. Symptoms may be present for several years before diagnosis. There is evidence that brain abnormalities are present for up to 30 years before symptoms are apparent so the true course of the disease is much longer.[9] Clearly, this presents an opportunity for interventions that could be applied before symptoms are apparent, providing accurate identification of pre-symptomatic Alzheimer's disease

were possible through a diagnostic test of blood, urine or cerebrospinal fluid (CSF). Such tests are otherwise known as 'peripheral biomarkers' of Alzheimer's disease because they do not involve direct testing of the central nervous system. There are already some exciting prospects on the horizon which are considered in Chapter 13.

Our understanding about what happens to the brain in Alzheimer's disease has increased dramatically in recent years, even if the precise reasons that cause the disease processes to commence are not fully understood. The genetic influences on the development of Alzheimer's disease are fully covered in Chapter 3 and are not repeated here.

As an overview, the Alzheimer's disease process initially destroys nerve cells in parts of the brain that control memory in the medial temporal lobe, including the hippocampus and related structures. With damage to the hippocampus, short-term memory fails impacting upon the person's daily function. Later the brain cortex, particularly the areas responsible for language and reasoning, becomes affected. Eventually, many other areas of the brain are involved and they atrophy (shrink) and lose function.[10, 11]

Senile (amyloid) plaques and the amyloid cascade hypothesis

As mentioned earlier, Alzheimer was the first to describe senile plaques. They consist of largely insoluble deposits of a type of protein known as beta-amyloid protein, and so they are sometimes called amyloid plaques. Beta-amyloid protein is derived from a larger protein called amyloid precursor protein (APP). The beta-amyloid aggregates or clumps together, and mixes with debris from neurons (nerve cells) and other cells to form the plaques. Although they can be found in normal older people, in Alzheimer's disease the plaques are predominantly found in areas of the brain used for memory and other cognitive functions – the hippocampus, medial temporal lobe and parietal lobe. Plaques are not likely to be the cause of the dementia; they are more likely to be a by-product of the disease process. Amyloid production, however, is central to the disease process.[12, 13]

John Hardy proposed the amyloid cascade hypothesis in the early 1990s after the discovery of mutations on the APP gene that were found to be associated with a rare form of younger-onset Alzheimer's disease. In essence, the amyloid cascade hypothesis states that amyloid deposits in Alzheimer's disease result from a number of genetic or environmental insults and lead to the degeneration of nerve cells that results in dementia. As beta-amyloid is derived from APP, a large protein with an unknown

function found throughout the brain, understanding the process by which it is produced from APP is of critical importance as it may provide a target for future treatments. APP is metabolised (broken down) by secretase enzymes in two distinct ways, one of which results in the formation of beta-amyloid. Both are normal processes, thus explaining why some plaques are found in normal people. The harmful pathway results in beta-amyloid being released into the space outside of the neuron where it begins to stick together in small soluble aggregates of beta-amyloid peptides called oligomers. These oligomers gradually clump together, becoming entities called fibrils, and along with other cellular material eventually form the insoluble amyloid plaques.[14]

In the rare familial younger-onset Alzheimer's disease, there is overproduction of beta-amyloid and increased plaque formation. In late-onset Alzheimer's disease, while there is normal production of beta-amyloid, there is a failure to degrade it which results in plaque formation. This implies that two basic therapeutic approaches could be applied – firstly, inhibit the production of beta-amyloid; secondly, promote the degradation of beta-amyloid.[15] However, it is unclear whether removal of beta-amyloid plaques will result in any improvement in mental function. As described in Chapter 13 research into these approaches is currently underway.

How does amyloid cause neurodegeneration?

In describing the disease process, I so far have made little mention of damage to nerve cells, which clearly has to occur for dementia to develop. Alzheimer's disease is characterised by abnormal cell death of vulnerable nerve cells in regions of the brain that are essential to normal cognitive function. It is this cell death that results in the brain atrophy, detectable on brain scans, so characteristic of the disease. The soluble beta-amyloid oligomers appear to cause the cell damage rather than the insoluble plaques. The oligomers react with neighbouring cells and synapses, disrupting their function. Beta-amyloid may increase 'programmed cell death' in the brain, an essentially normal process that helps weed out unnecessary or diseased cells, but which in the adult brain may result in irreversible loss of brain cells and function.[16]

Neurofibrillary tangles and tau protein

The second feature of Alzheimer's disease originally described by Alzheimer is the neurofibrillary tangle. Neurofibrillary tangles (NFTs) are

composed of a protein called tau. They are found in other degenerative disorders such as frontotemporal dementia. In contrast to plaques, the number of NFTs found in the brain and their anatomical localisation are strongly associated with the severity of dementia. Further, the NFTs are contained within the nerve cells and there is strong evidence to show that their presence heralds cell death. Thus there is strong circumstantial evidence that NFTs are essential components of the process that results in dementia. Tau protein normally stabilises microtubules in the neuron that are essential for the fast transport of microscopic components through the nerve cell. Damage to the microtubules disrupts the internal transport network of the neuron resulting in impairment of the ability of neurons to communicate with each other. In Alzheimer's disease, tau protein loses its ability to promote microtubule assembly and forms into NFTs.[17, 18]

This is a controversial area and for many years there have been two schools of thought about whether amyloid deposition or NFTs are the fundamental cause of Alzheimer's disease. (Humorists have labelled the two schools as BAPtists, for Beta-Amyloid Protein, and TAUists.) Certainly most evidence points to beta-amyloid as being the initial abnormality with NFT formation coming later. As in most complex systems, however, it is likely that both are critical to the disease process.

Neurotransmitters

Neurons communicate with each other by secreting chemicals known as neurotransmitters that bridge the microscopic gap between nerve cells at a point called the synapse. This is a complicated process that involves numerous steps, each of which may either inhibit or enhance the communication. There are numerous neurotransmitters in the brain including serotonin, noradrenaline, dopamine, glutamate and acetylcholine. In Alzheimer's disease, it has long been established that neurons secreting acetylcholine are the major ones affected by the disease.[19] Acetylcholine (cholinergic) pathways are critically important for normal memory function. It is not surprising that the initial recognition of the role of acetylcholine in Alzheimer's disease prompted trials of treatments to overcome the deficiency. After considerable early disappointment when efforts to directly boost the level of acetylcholine in the brain were ineffective, agents that indirectly boost the level of acetylcholine in the synapse by reducing its breakdown have been effective. These treatments are described in more detail in Chapter 7.

Many other neurotransmitters are affected in Alzheimer's disease, including glutamate that has an effect on learning; serotonin which affects mood and psychosis; gamma-aminobutyric acid (GABA) which has a role in anxiety and apathy; and noradrenaline, which is implicated with aggression.[20] Neurotransmitters also interact so that release of one neurotransmitter may have a modulating effect on another. An important issue to appreciate is that changes in neurotransmission in Alzheimer's disease only occur after there has been significant cell death. Acetylcholine deficiency is a result of the disease process, not a cause, so treatments that enhance the amount of acetylcholine in the brain are unlikely to alter the underlying disease process in a major way.

In summary, Alzheimer's disease is an age-related neurodegenerative disorder involving the clumping together of abnormal beta-amyloid and tau proteins in the brain over many years. This eventually results in a gradually progressive dementia due to neuronal dysfunction and cell death, particularly in the hippocampus, medial temporal and parietal lobes of the brain. Although there have been numerous risk factors identified as outlined in Chapters 2 and 3, most determine when the disease becomes symptomatic rather than being causal factors.

Vascular dementia

Some people believe that vascular dementia has been the 'forgotten' dementia, because of the degree of media attention about Alzheimer's disease. Further, the relative lack of research interest into treatments means that currently there is no cognitive enhancing drug proven to be effective in vascular dementia. Yet vascular dementia is the second most common type of dementia accounting for 20 to 30 per cent of cases, while perhaps 25 per cent of Alzheimer cases also have some vascular changes in the brain. It is more common in men than women in the general population. Vascular dementia is diagnosed when disease affecting blood vessels in the brain (cerebrovascular disease) is judged to be causal to the dementia. In contrast to Alzheimer's disease, a variety of processes is responsible for the dementia, and thus there is a wide range of clinical presentations.

Historically, vascular dementia has been described under a number of different terms. In the 19th century, 'arteriosclerotic dementia' was a term commonly used for what today would be mainly diagnosed as Alzheimer's disease. It was also recognised that apoplexy (stroke) often resulted in permanent changes in mental function, when the term 'post-apoplectic

dementia' was used. Following the better delineation of Alzheimer's disease, Vladimir Hachinski coined the term 'multi-infarct dementia' in 1974 to describe the dementia that results from multiple cerebral infarcts (strokes). As there are forms of dementia caused by cerebrovascular disease that are not due to multiple infarcts, the term vascular dementia was introduced in the 1990s as an umbrella term.[21]

Vascular dementia may result from single or multiple causes. The main causes are haemodynamic (blood flow to the brain) disorders (for example, strokes), thromboembolism (small blood clots originating mainly from the carotid artery or heart that block small blood vessels in the brain), small blood vessel disease in the brain (which results in a gradual reduction in blood supply to the brain), and haemorrhage (bleeding) into or around the brain (subarachnoid, intracerebral or subdural). Dementia following stroke is particularly common occurring in one quarter to one third of stroke victims, particularly when certain strategic areas of the brain are affected such as the frontal subcortical regions. Some researchers also hypothesise that stroke victims who develop dementia have early features of Alzheimer's disease that was not severe enough to cause symptoms before the stroke, but that reduce the brain reserve and leave the person vulnerable to the effects of the stroke. Prognosis is often poor as the risk of further stroke is high.[22, 23, 24]

Due to this range of causal disorders, the onset of symptoms in vascular dementia is quite variable, compared to Alzheimer's disease. Some symptoms may follow a sudden stroke, in other cases there may be a gradually progressive pattern with some fluctuation, in yet others there is the classic stepwise deterioration in which a sudden decline is followed by a period of stability before another sudden decline, and so on. To further complicate matters, some cases of vascular dementia are clinically almost indistinguishable from Alzheimer's disease, with gradual onset of slowly progressive cognitive impairment.

The Hachinski Scale was developed to help clinicians distinguish vascular dementia from Alzheimer's disease on clinical grounds. The items on the scale indicate clinical features that are more likely to occur in vascular dementia than in Alzheimer's disease. These include hypertension, depression, focal neurological symptoms (for example, limb paresis or weakness) or signs (for example, abnormal reflexes), sudden onset, and stepwise decline. Diagnosis of vascular dementia is aided by the demonstration of lesions caused by vascular disease on CT or MRI scans; in the absence of such findings, however, accurate differentiation

from Alzheimer's disease can be difficult if there has been an 'Alzheimer-type' onset. This difficulty is reflected in the lack of consensus between four internationally recognised sets of clinical diagnostic criteria for vascular dementia. Some clinicians tend to label all of these cases as 'mixed dementia', others as Alzheimer's disease. This is probably the major source of diagnostic inaccuracy in clinical dementia assessment.[25]

Because of this variety of pathologies responsible for the dementia, the clinical course of the disease is highly variable, though on the whole there is a worse prognosis than Alzheimer's disease. This may be due to the fact that people with vascular dementia are more likely to have serious cardiovascular disorders and other associated conditions including diabetes, hypertension, peripheral vascular disease and smoking-related disorders. Consequently, general medical management of the person with vascular dementia is of much greater importance than in Alzheimer's disease. Control of hypertension and diabetes, low-dose aspirin to reduce blood clotting, cessation of smoking, reduction of cholesterol, adequate exercise, low alcohol intake, weight control, stress management and low-fat/low-salt diet are all possible interventions.[26]

Dementia with Lewy bodies

Dementia with Lewy bodies (DLB) has only been recognised as a distinct entity since 1996 when consensus guidelines for the diagnosis first appeared.[27] It is estimated to account for about 5 per cent of dementia cases with around another 15 per cent occurring in combination with Alzheimer's disease.[28] For many years what is now known as DLB was felt to be a clinical subtype of Alzheimer's disease. This is one of the reasons that the delineation of the disorder has been so recent. It tends to occur in the age range of 50 to 85 years and is slightly more common in males. The mean duration of the disease is four and a half years, though it ranges from 1 to 20 years.[29]

The clinical features of DLB are quite striking. Onset of the disorder tends to be relatively sudden in comparison with Alzheimer's disease. The progressive cognitive decline is featured by poor attention and visuospatial function (ability of the brain to integrate visual and spatial information) but relatively intact memory. Cognition tends to fluctuate to the extent that the patient may appear to be in an acute confusional state; frequently, however, extensive hospital investigation fails to identify a cause. At other times fluctuating cognition may simply be mistaken for daytime

tiredness. Visual hallucinations are often prominent early in the course of the illness and usually involve animals or people – they are sometimes frightening but often not. Features of parkinsonism with muscular rigidity, tremors and slowed movements are common, but characteristically these develop alongside the cognitive changes. When Parkinson's disease has been present for a year or more before the dementia, it is more correctly diagnosed as Parkinson's disease dementia. Recurrent falls, faints that are often misdiagnosed as TIAs, depression and sensitivity to antipsychotic medication (often prescribed for the hallucinations) are features that support the diagnosis.[30]

Lewy bodies are found in neurons and contain the protein alpha-synuclein, which interferes with neuronal function. Friedrich Lewy, who worked in the same laboratory as Alzheimer, first described them in 1912. They have long been recognised as being the main brain abnormality of Parkinson's disease. Although regularly noted to be present in the cortical areas of brains of Alzheimer patients, until the early 1990s this was thought to be an incidental finding as the number present seemed insufficient to cause brain damage.[31]

At about this time new laboratory techniques resulted in the Lewy bodies being more easily seen under the microscope. Suddenly, researchers in Newcastle upon Tyne and San Diego in particular became aware that Lewy bodies were present in large amounts in the brains of up to 36 per cent of Alzheimer patients. Because Lewy bodies are so pale, they had been very difficult to see in cerebral white matter with standard stains used for the previous century. This quickly led to a re-evaluation of the clinical syndrome. Similar to Alzheimer's disease, there is a marked deficit in acetylcholine in the brain but there are also deficits of the neurotransmitter dopamine. The cholinergic deficits mean that the cholinesterase inhibitor drugs primarily designed for Alzheimer's disease are also beneficial in DLB, with some experience suggesting a better response than found in Alzheimer's disease.[32]

Frontotemporal dementia

Frontotemporal dementia is a term used to describe a group of neurodegenerative disorders that includes Pick's disease, a condition first described by Arnold Pick over a century ago. It accounts for approximately 5 to 10 per cent of dementia cases and is particularly common in younger age groups, usually developing between the ages of 35 and 75 years,

with no gender differences. Frontotemporal dementia primarily affects the frontal lobe (an area responsible for 'executive functions' such as reasoning, judgement, insight, personality, aspects of memory, and social behaviour) and the anterior temporal lobe (an area responsible for speech, language and aspects of memory) of the brain. Frontotemporal dementia runs a course of between two and ten years after diagnosis.[33]

In 20 to 40 per cent of cases there is a family history of dementia but, as noted in Chapter 3, true familial forms only account for around 10 to 15 per cent of cases. A simple definition is where there are two or more family members with the condition at a younger age of onset (often loosely defined as under 65 years of age).

One major similarity to Alzheimer's disease is the characteristic accumulation of abnormal tau protein inside nerve cells in neurofibrillary tangles, disrupting normal nerve cell processes and ultimately leading to cell death. Other changes include a progressive loss of nerve cells in the frontal and temporal regions of the brain, gliosis (nerve tissue scarring) and vacuolation, a process in which 'holes' form in the outer layer of the brain. In Pick's disease, characteristic Pick bodies are found in neurons.

Frontotemporal dementia has an insidious onset. There are two main clinical types which are determined by the area of the brain that is primarily affected. *Behavioural-variant frontotemporal dementia* occurs when mainly the frontal lobe is involved and in this condition the predominant initial features are behaviour and personality changes, including loss of emotional warmth, selfishness, apathy, altered eating behaviour, socially and sexually inappropriate behaviours, irritability, compulsive behaviours, usually accompanied by loss of awareness or concern about the behaviour change.[34]

Semantic dementia occurs when the temporal lobe is mainly involved and this usually presents with a decline in language function in which the meaning of words is affected. Commonly the initial complaint is of being unable to remember words including people's names but as the disease progresses there is loss of spontaneous speech (often interpreted by family members as being due to lack of interest or depression), speech comprehension is impaired, reading and spelling are affected and eventually, as the frontal lobes become affected, behaviour changes too.[35] Another rarer type of speech impairment occurs in *progressive non-fluent aphasia* and involves stuttering with frequent paraphasic errors where the wrong word is used (for example, saying that a comb is a brush), the use of

non-grammatical speech and stereotypical speech where the same words, phrases or themes are repeated.[36]

With behavioural and personality changes it can be some years before it becomes apparent that there may be an underlying brain disorder. This is particularly the case in a younger person, where problems may initially be attributed to such diverse issues as work stress, depression, alcohol or drug abuse, marital disharmony or the menopause. Eventually memory and language impairment become more obvious. People with frontotemporal dementia may also develop motor difficulties like those seen in Parkinson's disease. These include muscle rigidity, lack of balance and stiffness of movement, but not the limb tremors at rest that are characteristic of Parkinson's.

The diagnostic assessment of people with suspected frontotemporal dementia usually requires a neuropsychological evaluation as part of the dementia work up as many of the standard cognitive tests used in routine dementia assessment are relatively insensitive to impaired frontal lobe function. At times even the initial neuropsychological evaluation will be equivocal and repeat testing 6 to 12 months later may be necessary. One major difference between frontotemporal dementia and Alzheimer's disease is that people with frontotemporal dementia do not suffer as much memory loss, tend to know where they are, and are able to recall information about the past and present. Even in the late stages, people with frontotemporal dementia, unlike those with Alzheimer's disease, are able to negotiate their surroundings and remain well oriented.[37]

Currently there are no specific treatments available that can slow or stop the disease process. Other general treatments for some of the symptoms and behaviours are covered in Chapter 7.

Other neurodegenerative causes of dementia

Parkinson's disease characteristically presents with tremors, slowing of limb movements and increased muscle tone or stiffness. A shuffling style of walking with a stooped posture and lack of arm swing is common. Dementia develops later in the course of the disease. Parkinson's disease that develops in late life has a high risk of progressing to dementia with features that are often similar to dementia with Lewy bodies.

A range of other less common neurodegenerative disorders also cause dementia. *Corticobasal degeneration* and *progressive supranuclear palsy* are related to frontotemporal dementia inasmuch as they are caused by tau protein aggregation in neurons.[38] Corticobasal degeneration has

symptoms that often appear to be a mix of Parkinson's and Alzheimer's disease. Progressive supranuclear palsy, the disease from which the English comedian Dudley Moore died, mainly involves the brainstem and areas known as the basal ganglia. The clinical features include those of Parkinson's disease, instability when standing and walking (the sufferer may appear 'intoxicated' and have falls), and difficulties in looking upwards with the eyes.

Creutzfeldt-Jakob disease (CJD) is a prion disease. Prions are small glycoproteins with infectious qualities that cause amyloid formation and nerve degeneration. CJD is characterised by a rapidly progressive dementia (death usually within two years) with features of muscular jerks (myoclonus), and unsteadiness of gait and neurological features implying involvement of the cortical and subcortical structures of the brain. Although most attention has been given in the popular press to infectious forms, particularly that associated with bovine spongiform encephalopathy (BSE or mad cow disease), there is also a very rare inherited form that accounts for between 5 and 10 per cent of cases. A mutation on the PRioN Protein (PRNP) gene accounts for 70 per cent of the inherited form of CJD worldwide.[39]

Huntington's disease is a genetic disorder with abnormalities on chromosome 4. All carriers of the gene will get the disease and children of carriers have a 50 per cent chance of getting it. It is a neurodegenerative disorder characterised by abnormal involuntary movements of the body (choreiform movements), personality change, and psychiatric problems that usually pre-date the process of the dementia. It usually has an age of onset between 30 and 45 years but cases outside of this age range also occur. Sporadic cases without a known family history can also occur.

Familial British dementia (FBD) is a rare disease characterised by progressive dementia, paralysis, and loss of balance. It usually occurs around age 40 to 50. Similar to Alzheimer's disease, FBD patients have amyloid deposition associated with blood vessels and NFTs.[40] It is due to a defect in the gene called BRI, which is located on chromosome 13. A close variant of the disorder was found in a small Danish population.[41]

Secondary dementias

Some of the other less common types of dementia are potentially reversible and are the focus of investigations during dementia assessment as described in Chapter 6. They are more likely to be found in younger-onset dementia. These include neurosyphilis (the late stage of untreated

syphilis that may occur many years after the initial venereal infection), disorders of the thyroid gland, deficiencies of vitamin B_{12} and folic acid, chronic drug intoxication, chronic meningitis, cerebral vasculitis due to autoimmune disorders such as temporal arteritis and various metabolic disorders.[42]

Normal pressure hydrocephalus is a condition in which an intermittent blockage of the flow of cerebrospinal fluid (CSF) around the brain can result in marked dilatation of the cerebral ventricles (cistern-like structures inside the brain) through build-up of the CSF and subsequent compression and death of brain tissue. The early symptoms are gait disturbances, incontinence of urine and confusion, usually developing over a few months. It tends to occur in younger people (most commonly 40 to 70 years of age) and is predisposed by a history of meningitis, subarachnoid haemorrhage, head trauma or cerebral tumours, although in nearly 50 per cent of cases there is no known cause. After it was first described in the 1960s, many dementia patients who had a gait disturbance, urinary incontinence and were found to have large cerebral ventricles on brain scan, had neurosurgery in which a shunt was placed into the brain to drain away the excess CSF. Approximately 50 per cent of patients improved, usually those people whose symptoms had developed in the previous few months, had a known cause for the condition and did not have signs of brain atrophy on scans. It became clear that many of those operated upon, particularly those with dementia symptoms for over six months and without any other obvious cause for the dilatation of the cerebral ventricles, did not have normal pressure hydrocephalus. Indeed, they were mainly Alzheimer patients. Furthermore, there were frequent surgical complications especially infections of the implanted shunts that necessitated repeated procedures.[43] Normal pressure hydrocephalus is infrequently diagnosed now but new interest has been expressed about the use of shunts as a treatment for Alzheimer's disease (see Chapter 13).

Alcohol-related dementia (ARD) is a somewhat controversial diagnosis as there is debate about whether it is a distinct clinical entity and about what relationship it has with Wernicke-Korsakoff syndrome. It is clear that alcohol abuse and associated thiamine deficiency can cause Wernicke-Korsakoff syndrome which has well-documented neuropathology resulting in profound chronic short-term memory impairment and executive dysfunction resulting in behavioural and personality change. What is less clear is whether alcohol neurotoxicity alone results in dementia and what the actual neuropathology is. In autopsy studies of the brains of

people diagnosed with ARD, many cases are found to have either vascular dementia or Alzheimer's disease although one study has reported synapse loss in frontal cortical regions similar to those seen in frontotemporal dementia and other studies have found evidence of thiamine deficiency too. It seems likely that there is overlap between ARD and Wernicke-Korsakoff syndrome. It remains a diagnosis that is frequently used in areas with high rates of alcohol abuse and is particularly common in younger-onset dementia. What is most important is that ARD is potentially preventable with abstinence from alcohol and adequate thiamine replacement.[44]

Head injuries that cause dementia are usually very severe, and it may be some months before sufficient recovery from the acute confusion has occurred to determine what deficits remain. One characteristic of the dementia is that improvement may continue for some years after the injury. Another is that in those who recover, a delayed onset of dementia may occur some years later as indicated by head injury being a risk factor for Alzheimer's disease.

Brain tumours are discovered quite frequently in dementia investigation. Most are small inconsequential benign meningiomas that have little effect and don't require treatment. Some are large enough and located at a site to warrant surgical removal. In my experience, this rarely results in cognitive improvement, but may prevent further decline. Occasionally malignant tumours such as gliomas may cause dementia, and here the prognosis is very poor.

AIDS dementia complex (ADC), otherwise known as *HIV-associated dementia (HAD)*, occurs in up to 15 per cent of HIV-infected adults. In over 90 per cent of cases it develops in the last year of life. Unlike other AIDS-defining illnesses, the standard highly active antiretroviral therapy (HAART) has not had much impact on the development of ADC, possibly due to poor central nervous system penetration. Therapy has also been limited by an incomplete understanding of how ADC occurs. Central nervous system infection might be present in persons with otherwise early stable HIV infection raising the prospect that HAART may be required earlier than currently used in standard approaches to HIV treatment in order to prevent dementia. There is an absence of large, adequate and well-controlled clinical trials using agents that protect nerve cells or those with disease-modifying potential. In general, people with ADC have little involvement with mainstream dementia services. This is in part due to their average age of around 35 years, although HIV-infected persons have had increased life expectancy in recent years that approaches that of

the general population. Another factor is the stigma attached to the term 'dementia' that is associated with old age and Alzheimer's disease.[45, 46, 47]

Summary

Apart from vascular dementia, most common types of dementia including Alzheimer's disease are caused by the gradual abnormal accumulation of toxic proteins in the brain that results in neurodegeneration, in turn resulting in impaired neuronal function and cell death.

Dementia Assessment

'Am I getting dementia?' Some people ask this question because they have noticed a change in their memory. There are many reasons that older people acquire symptoms that may raise fears within themselves, in their family, their friends or their doctors about the possibility that they are developing dementia. Subjective memory concerns are frequently due to self-awareness of normal age-related cognitive change, anxiety, depression and various medical problems such as thyroid underactivity.

> *Carmel had always been a 'worrier'; now at the age of 70 she was concerned that her memory was failing. She complained to her doctor that she kept forgetting the reason that she had gone from one room to another in her home, but admitted that after some minutes it would usually come back to her. She couldn't recall the details of conversations she had with her husband and friends, though she remembered having the conversations. And, of course, she could never remember people's names and that was so embarrassing! Recently, she had felt under some stress. Her older daughter had divorced, her husband had suffered a heart attack though was now well, and a good friend had died.*

It is important to get a basic check-up with your doctor if you are in this situation as there may be a simple explanation for what you have noticed which will respond to treatment. If there is no simple explanation, a formal dementia assessment may be called for. This assessment aims to determine the cause of these symptoms and to recommend appropriate management.

What is dementia assessment?

The precise components of the assessment process for dementia will vary according to the nature of the presenting symptoms and the centre where

it is undertaken, but there are a number of basic principles. As noted in Chapter 4, early symptoms of dementia may be subtle and equivocal. In this circumstance, the initial focus will be to determine whether or not the problem is caused by dementia or some other condition. On the other hand, many people still present for assessment with symptoms of well-established dementia and here the main focus will be more on establishing the type of dementia. In either circumstance, dementia assessment includes all aspects of the gathering of information about a person that enables an accurate identification of the symptoms – description of behaviours, identification of psychosocial issues, measurement of functional capacity, and determination of relevant medical conditions (which will certainly include a range of diagnostic investigations). An adequate assessment requires the involvement of the person's spouse, children, siblings, friends and occasionally parents to corroborate information, to provide additional details from an observer perspective and usually to allow an assessment of their needs as caregivers or potential caregivers.

Who should perform the assessment?

Initial assessment – screening

A range of assessment options is available in most places. Ideally, the person's local doctor or their practice nurse should undertake the initial assessment but other possibilities include a community aged care service or, if the person is in hospital for some reason, hospital doctors and nurses. In each of these settings, it is commonplace these days for a routine screening examination to be performed on all older patients, especially those aged over 75.

Screening involves a brief examination of mental function to determine whether there are signs of possible dementia or another mental and/or physical disorder. Most doctors have been taught how to use at least one of a number of 'screening tests' for cognitive function that take 5–10 minutes to complete. Examples include the Abbreviated Mental Test Score (AMTS),[1] the Rowland Universal Dementia Assessment Scale (RUDAS),[2] the Mini Mental State Examination (MMSE),[3] and the General Practitioner Assessment of Cognition (GPCOG).[4] Each of these tests has in common questions that check the person's immediate memory and short-term memory in a standardised fashion. For example, being able to recall either a set of words or a name and address both immediately and after about three minutes is used to check memory function. Other cognitive functions are covered to varying degrees in the different tests.

The tests are standardised, so the scores obtained give an indication as to whether there is likely to be a significant impairment of cognitive function requiring a more substantial examination. On the MMSE, the 'cut-off' score is 24 out of 30 and on the AMTS it is 7 out of 10. This doesn't mean that a score below the cut-off scores equates with dementia.[5, 6] A person who is severely depressed or moribund with an infection may score well below the cut-off scores when unwell but well above when recovered. Other factors that may lower scores include poor education, poor hearing, limited English language skills, life-long developmental delay and severe psychiatric disorders such as schizophrenia. The RUDAS was developed in Australia for use in people from culturally and linguistically diverse backgrounds and has been shown to perform as well as the MMSE but without some of the culturally inappropriate and education-influenced items found in the latter scale.[7]

Some people with early dementia will score above the cut-off. This is more likely to occur in an intelligent person who may have declined from their pre-morbid level of cognitive function but not sufficiently to be detected by the screen. Thus, to improve the chances of detecting a clinically significant problem, it is advisable for the doctor or nurse to obtain collateral information from the person's partner, friends or family. The advantage of the GPCOG, developed in Australia by Professor Henry Brodaty and colleagues, is that it includes some questions to elicit such information as part of the standardised scale. Further assessment would be warranted if informants had noticed a decline even if the screening test was above the cut-off score, particularly if it was just above the cut-off or if some points had been lost on the short-term memory task. A free online version is now available (see Appendix 2).[8]

This initial assessment, when allied with a general check-up, should identify most persons likely to have early dementia and these require a more thorough examination. Others will have been found to be anxious, depressed or have some other medical problem as described later that is responsible for the symptoms. This group should have these problems treated and have their cognition reviewed when they have fully recovered. A third group has symptoms that do not appear to be significant – they score above the cut-offs on the screening tests and their informants haven't noticed much change. In most cases it would be reasonable to take a 'wait-and-see' approach by reviewing the situation every six months. However, if the doctor, patient or patient's family were uneasy with this, it would be wise to seek a specialist opinion.

Definitive assessment

A definitive assessment should contain a number of components that are listed in Box 6.1.

Box 6.1 Domains of definitive dementia assessment

- Full history, full mental state examination (including cognitive assessment with a reliable standardised scale) and physical examination by an appropriately trained medical practitioner.

- Collateral history from support person (partner, sibling, child, friend) to obtain a description of the cognitive, behavioural and functional changes in addition to medical history.

- Identification of psychosocial issues including any potential relationship difficulties between the person with dementia and their main supports, caregiver concerns and stress, financial circumstances, knowledge/fears about dementia.

- Measurement of functional capacity including work, driving, financial competency (power of attorney, will).

- Appropriate laboratory, radiological and other investigations as required to establish the correct diagnosis.

These combine:

- to construct a prioritised problem list

- to determine the cause of the cognitive change

- to devise a management plan with the patient and their supporters that includes:

  - explanation of the diagnosis or further action required to determine the diagnosis

  - dementia education and information about appropriate services including the Alzheimer's Association

  - treatment options

  - planning for the future – wills, financial management, driving competency

  - answering any questions about the diagnosis

  - follow-up arrangements.

Table 6.1 Dementia investigations

Routine investigations	Reason(s) for the investigation
Full (complete) blood count	To exclude anaemia, infections
Urea, creatinine and electrolytes	To exclude kidney and metabolic disorders
Calcium	To exclude high calcium e.g. due to tumours
Liver function tests	To exclude liver failure, liver tumours
Serum vitamin B_{12} and red blood cell folate	To exclude deficiency states, pernicious anaemia
Erythrocyte Sedimentation Rate (ESR), C-reactive protein (CRP)	Often abnormal when inflammatory conditions such as vasculitis and infections are present
Thyroid function tests	To exclude overactive and underactive thyroid gland
Fasting serum homocysteine	To exclude CNS B-group vitamin/folate deficiency
Brain CT scan	To exclude strokes, tumours, subdural haematomas and hydrocephalus and to determine whether brain atrophy is present

Investigations required when clinically indicated

Neuropsychological examination	To distinguish mild cognitive impairment from early dementia and to assist in diagnosing the type of dementia
Brain MRI scan	To exclude vasculitis or encephalopathy and to obtain higher resolution brain images, particularly of the hippocampus
Chest X-ray	To exclude tumours and infections
Electrocardiogram (ECG)	To exclude cardiac causes of vascular dementia
Holter monitor	To exclude cardiac causes of vascular dementia

cont.

Routine investigations	Reason(s) for the investigation
Carotid dopplers	To exclude carotid artery disease as a cause of vascular dementia
Echocardiogram	To exclude cardiac causes of vascular dementia
Fasting blood sugar level	To exclude diabetes mellitus
Syphilis serology	To exclude syphilis infection
Human Immunodeficiency Virus (HIV) screen	To exclude HIV/AIDS-related disorder
Immunological screen	To exclude autoimmune disorders
Microurine	To exclude urinary infections and renal disease
Electroencephalogram (EEG)	To exclude epilepsy and encephalopathy
Lumbar puncture	To exclude meningitis or encephalitis
Sleep studies	To exclude sleep apnea
SPECT, PET or PiB scan	To assist in the diagnosis of early Alzheimer's disease and clarify specific type of dementia in select cases
Genetic screening	For those at risk of familial forms of dementia
APOE testing	To determine if APOE ε4 allele is present indicating higher risk of Alzheimer's disease – not recommended in routine dementia investigation

Once it has been determined that a more thorough assessment is required, this almost certainly means an examination by a medical specialist – psychiatrist, neurologist or geriatrician depending on local availability and the type of presenting symptoms. For example, it may be best for a person who is depressed with memory loss to see a psychiatrist, either an old age psychiatrist (geriatric psychiatrist, psychogeriatrician) or neuropsychiatrist. It may be best for an aged person with multiple medical problems and confusion to see a geriatrician. Neurologists might be the most appropriate

specialists to see younger persons with cognitive impairment, persons with rapidly progressive cognitive change, or persons with other neurological symptoms such as gait problems. This does not necessarily mean an immediate referral. Many local doctors will quite appropriately do a more detailed examination and undertake the routine investigations described in Table 6.1 before referral.[9] Frequently local doctors will determine the correct diagnosis but most will prefer to have this confirmed by a specialist. In Australia, the Pharmaceutical Benefit Scheme (PBS) regulations for prescribing subsidised cholinesterase inhibitor drugs for Alzheimer's disease require a specialist confirmation of Alzheimer's disease.

Memory clinics that specialise in dementia assessment are another option. The advantages of memory clinics are that they are thorough and are usually multidisciplinary. Most of them routinely engage neuropsychologists for a detailed cognitive assessment, social workers to assess the family circumstances, occupational therapists to determine the person's level of function and community nurses in addition to one or more of the medical specialists previously mentioned (see Box 6.2). Usually there is an assessment protocol that involves examination by the various health professionals over a number of sessions spread over a few weeks. The protocol includes the various diagnostic investigations required to make an accurate dementia diagnosis. The final diagnosis and management recommendations are often determined by consensus opinion from the various team members.

Memory clinics may not be suitable for all cases of suspected dementia. They are probably most useful in suspected early dementia and where there are no major associated medical or psychological problems. A geriatrician and multidisciplinary aged care team may better assess frail, older people, and those with more severe cognitive impairment of long standing, in the person's home. Similarly, old age mental health services would be better placed to see depressed or psychotic persons with suspected dementia. Usually assessments by these other services will include many of the multidisciplinary assessments that take place in memory clinics but are more likely to be tailored to the individual case. For example, many with mild dementia and most with moderate-severe dementia will not require a full neuropsychological examination.

Box 6.2 Components of multidisciplinary dementia assessment

Medical assessment

This involves a full medical history, mental state examination and physical examination. The history is usually obtained from both the cognitively impaired person and the primary informant to enable a more accurate understanding of the problems. The mental state examination explores both cognitive and psychological functioning to determine the extent of cognitive deficits and whether there is a psychiatric disorder, especially depression, present. Standardised cognitive and depression scales are usually used. The physical examination focuses mainly on the neurological and vascular systems.

Neuropsychological assessment

This is a two to three-hour assessment performed by a trained neuropsychologist using a battery of standardised tests to evaluate cognitive functions in different parts of the brain. Test scores are compared with population norms; some tests are designed to enable an estimation of function before the onset of disease. They are particularly useful in quantifying memory impairment and in determining the pattern of cognitive deficits that may help in determining the type of dementia. Where deficits are mild or equivocal, repeat testing in 12 to 18 months may identify changes not detected by other assessments. Neuropsychologists are usually only available in major centres.

Social work assessment

There are two basic strands to this assessment. One focuses on the social function and support network of the person with dementia and attempts to determine whether any additional social supports are required. The other focuses on the person with dementia's family and other caregivers, assessing their level of stress and how well they are coping. In some centres, this latter assessment may be linked with caregiver support groups. The social worker will often be responsible for arranging whatever community services are determined to be necessary.

Occupational therapy assessment

This assessment is usually carried out in the home of the person with dementia. It aims to determine their functional capacity by assessing their ability to perform various activities of daily living. In those with mild cognitive impairments, the assessment concentrates on higher-order activities such as financial management, meal preparation, telephone use and organisational skills. Driving assessments may be undertaken as a separate task, usually in a specialised centre. Where there are more severe deficits, more basic skills such as dressing, bathing and toileting are covered. An assessment of the home for basic safety is also done – for example, if the person has a history of falls, recommendations might be made about the installation of rails.

Nursing assessment

In many centres, community nurses perform a combination of cognitive screening, health screening, assessment of social needs, and functional assessments. This is especially the case where the nurse is part of a community aged care team. Medication management is a common issue that requires assessment in those who live alone.

It is not essential that all these assessments be undertaken in every case during the initial assessment process. For example, in mild cognitive impairment it may not be necessary to have an occupational therapy assessment, as there are few relevant deficits. Also, many doctors give sufficient time to family members to talk over their concerns and if they are coping without significant problems, a social work assessment may not be required. These other assessments can then be undertaken at a later point if the situation changes.

What else may be causing memory changes? The differential diagnosis of dementia

Throughout the assessment process, the aim is to eliminate any other condition as the cause of the person's cognitive impairment before determining the type of dementia. The main conditions that need to be excluded are described here.

Depression

In Chapter 4, I demonstrated how depression might be the forerunner of dementia. There are also situations where depression may mimic dementia. After the age of 40, most people who are clinically depressed probably have some degree of memory impairment. Such impairments are more noticeable with increasing age and severity of the depression. Occasionally, the effects upon memory function can be so severe that the person may seem, superficially at least, to be suffering from dementia, which led to the coining of the term 'pseudodementia'. Other psychiatric disorders such as schizophrenia and anxiety may also cause pseudodementia, but depression is the most common cause.

The classic depressive pseudodementia is caused by a severe major depression, and although the cognitive impairment resolves with treatment of the depression, there is a high relapse rate and in many cases the cognitive impairment may not fully resolve. Sometimes the residual

impairment is age-related and benign, at other times it may be due to coexisting brain disease such as stroke or Parkinson's disease. Furthermore, while in persons under 60 the risk for the later development of dementia is no higher than for other people who have an episode of depression (see Chapter 3), in people older than 60, approximately 25 to 50 per cent develop dementia within three to five years.[10]

The late Foundation Professor of Psychiatry at the University of NSW in Sydney, Leslie Kiloh, wrote the seminal paper on pseudodementia in 1961. He stressed that in these patients depression could closely mimic the appearance of dementia to the extent that the treatment of depression could be neglected. He cautioned clinicians to consider the possibility of depression whenever the diagnosis of dementia was being considered.[11]

To fully understand the historical context, it needs to be appreciated that in the early 1960s all cases of dementia were considered irreversible. Senile dementia was regarded as either a normal part of ageing or due to arteriosclerosis ('hardening of the arteries'), and thus investigation of the cause was not routinely undertaken except in younger people. Consequently, the prospect of older people with undiagnosed depression left lingering untreated in an asylum, because they had been mistakenly diagnosed with dementia, was not far-fetched. Today this would be an extremely unlikely circumstance due to the better education of health professionals and the community, and the assessment process that occurs if people are being considered for admission into long-term residential care.

A more common situation that prevails today concerns the person diagnosed with dementia complicated by depression, where it is uncertain how much depression is causing the symptoms (and hence potentially amenable to antidepressant therapy) and how much is due to dementia. This raises questions about how far trials of treatment should go. Sometimes there is no clear answer to the therapeutic dilemma.[12] This is discussed in more detail in Chapter 7.

'Reversible' causes of dementia

With the recognition that depression and normal pressure hydrocephalus could present, albeit only occasionally, in a similar fashion to typical cases of senile dementia, researchers around the world began to conduct thorough investigations of patients referred to specialist centres for assessment of dementia or memory impairment. Numerous studies in the 1970s and 1980s reported that up to 17 per cent of people referred for assessment of dementia had potentially reversible conditions. These studies have been

very influential on current clinical practice – the ubiquitous 'dementia screen' of investigations outlined in Table 6.1 was derived from them.

I published a systematic review of these studies in 1991 and concluded that while there were many medical disorders that caused cognitive impairment, most reported cases failed to meet the diagnostic criteria for dementia. Those which did meet the criteria for dementia infrequently recovered. Improvements in mental function generally occurred when diagnostic criteria for dementia were not met, the duration of symptoms was less than six months, and when there was only a mild degree of cognitive impairment. Only 3 per cent of patients fully recovered; of these about two thirds were either depressed or affected by prescription drugs, usually psychotropic medication. These conditions were diagnosed clinically rather than by investigations. Indeed, in only 5 per cent of all cases assessed did investigations discover treatable conditions that resulted in cognitive improvement.[13]

Most people with 'reversible dementia' do not actually have dementia. The correct diagnostic terminology would in many cases be delirium, which is a global disorder of cognition that develops over days to weeks and is characterised by fluctuations in alertness, changes in the sleep–wake cycle, poor concentration and memory, visual hallucinations and motor changes of restlessness or apathy. It is when a sub-acute delirium develops over weeks to a few months that a dementia-like state can occur, which could be due to the gradual accumulation of drugs such as antidepressants, sedatives and anticonvulsants, for example. The effects of drug accumulation might be manifested as a sleep disorder such as sleep apnea. When alcohol abuse is the cause of cognitive impairment, cessation of drinking together with thiamine supplements often results in improved cognition.

This does not mean the investigations are unnecessary – they are essential in obtaining an accurate diagnosis; frequently, coincidental medical disorders are discovered that require treatment. Table 6.1 summarises the investigations that are essential and those that are used in select cases. Brain scans allow the clinician to view the brain in three dimensions and see its internal structures. There are many types of brain scans, with the most commonly used one being the Computerised Tomography (CT) scan which is inexpensive and available in most parts of the world. It takes around 20 minutes to complete and most people with dementia are able to tolerate it. Some clinicians prefer a Magnetic Resonance Imaging (MRI) brain scan instead of a CT scan as a MRI provides better-quality images, especially if very small lesions are expected, for example little strokes.

It also allows clearer images of the hippocampus, an important structure in Alzheimer's disease. However, in most cases an MRI is not essential. It is more expensive than a CT scan, has more limited availability, and in some countries requires a specialist referral. As it involves lying in an enclosed cylinder, it can aggravate claustrophobia and some people become quite frightened with the procedure. People with cardiac pacemakers or other metallic implants are unable to have MRI scans due to the effects of the magnetism on their implants.

Other investigations do not have any routine clinical role and have been mainly used in research settings. Examples include positron emission tomography (PET) scans and single photon emission computed tomography (SPECT) scans that are used to measure brain function and the Pittsburgh-B compound (PiB) PET scan which measures the amount of amyloid protein in the brain and might facilitate the earlier diagnosis of Alzheimer's disease. These are described in more detail in Chapter 13. Genetic screening is only usually performed in persons with a strong family history of dementia at a younger age.

Normal ageing

While it may seem strange to include normality within the differential diagnosis of dementia, this is not too uncommon a finding in older people referred for dementia assessment. The typical 'normal' older person who is referred (usually at their own insistence) for dementia assessment is a rather anxious individual who is well informed about Alzheimer's disease and has become aware of changes in their memory function and fears the worst. When a thorough examination reveals that they are functioning normally, albeit in a manner tainted by anxiety, reassurance that their mental function is normal often suffices. Of course, one can never be absolute in such reassurance, and I usually suggest that they return for a check-up in 12 months, for there is a fine line between normality and mild cognitive impairment, particularly within older age groups.

Mild cognitive impairment

Most people with Alzheimer's disease experience a subtle cognitive decline before reaching the clinical threshold of symptoms that enables diagnosis. Mild cognitive impairment (MCI) refers to this transitional state between normal ageing and mild dementia. This condition has only been characterised in the past decade, so relatively little is known about it and there is still scientific debate about its validity.

Most research to date has focused on those individuals who present with a subjective memory complaint and have an objective memory impairment compared with normal persons of the same age and educational background. While not essential to the diagnosis, it is preferable for the change in cognitive function to be corroborated by an informant. People with MCI have preserved activities of daily living, but it does appear that higher-order instrumental activities that require greater cognitive input are likely to be mildly impaired. Although memory impairment is frequently the main and only concern (amnestic MCI), other cognitive domains can be affected too. When multiple cognitive domains including memory are affected (multidomain amnestic MCI), there is a higher risk of conversion to dementia. Persons diagnosed with MCI will need to be reviewed at least annually and at these times have repeat cognitive testing and possibly repeat CT/MRI scans to determine if there is any progressive atrophy, particularly around the hippocampus.[14]

Focal brain syndromes

Focal brain syndromes occur when only a discrete part of the brain is damaged. They are distinct from dementia because they lack the global disturbances of brain function and are not usually progressive. They can often be severely disabling in their own right, however, and at times the distinction will not alter many aspects of the person's capacity or the type of care required.

Amnestic syndromes are mainly characterised by profound impairments of short-term memory without other cognitive changes. The most frequently cited cause of amnestic syndrome is Wernicke-Korsakoff disorder that is due to thiamine deficiency damaging the hippocampus, a part of the brain critical for short-term memory function. Alcohol abuse is the commonest cause of the Wernicke-Korsakoff syndrome with other causes including gastric stapling, hunger strikes and prolonged intravenous therapy without thiamine supplementation. Most cases due to alcohol are not considered 'pure' amnestic syndromes insofar as alcohol also damages the frontal lobe of the brain, which means that it is not focal damage and is really consistent with dementia. Often the term 'alcohol-related brain damage' is used to reflect this combination of disorders thus avoiding the diagnosis of dementia but it is applied inconsistently by clinicians (see Chapter 5).[15] Other causes of amnestic syndrome include pituitary tumours, carbon monoxide poisoning, herpes simplex encephalitis and brain trauma.

Frontal lobe syndromes from damage to the frontal lobe of the brain commonly occur due to excessive alcohol intake (three or more standard drinks per day in a woman, four or more in a man) but are also caused by brain tumours (particularly meningiomas), strokes and subdural haematomas (blood clots) located in this region. Frontal lobe damage is liable to result in behavioural changes; the precise pattern of symptoms will depend on the part of the frontal lobe involved. There are three general patterns: an apathetic, dulled, unmotivated, depressive pattern; a disinhibited, jocular, childlike pattern with poor self-control; and a pattern with poor organisational and planning skills and impaired abstract conceptualisation. Impaired insight and judgement occur to some extent in all three patterns.

Treatment of the cause of the focal brain syndrome usually results in a stable but unremitting impairment. Severely disabled individuals may require long-term residential care, while the moderately impaired usually need some level of ongoing external support from family, friends and community services.

Making the diagnosis

The diagnosis of dementia should be based on well-established diagnostic criteria with information obtained in the clinical examination. Once the dementia diagnosis has been made, the type of dementia needs to be determined and here, investigations may identify some concurrent disorder, for example, stroke or thyroid deficiency. Currently there is no available test (blood, urine, CSF or neuroimaging) that can confirm the diagnosis of Alzheimer's disease, though some have been promoted from time to time. In the 1990s, a pupillary dilation test was promoted as being diagnostic for Alzheimer's disease but this proved to be incorrect. There are future prospects for such tests, including the previously mentioned PiB PET scan, and these are discussed in Chapter 13.

Diagnostic criteria for Alzheimer's disease were first published by the US Alzheimer's Association and the National Institute of Neurological and Communicative Disorders and Stroke in 1984 with a revision published in 2011.[16] The Alzheimer's disease diagnosis is based on the presence of typical clinical features and the absence of other identifiable causes. The definitive diagnosis of Alzheimer's disease requires the demonstration of typical neuropathology in brain tissue. As this could only be obtained in life through brain biopsy, confirmation of the diagnosis usually only occurs at autopsy.

The convention is thus to use the term '*probable* Alzheimer's disease' where diagnostic criteria are met and all other possible causes of dementia are eliminated, and '*possible* Alzheimer's disease' where diagnostic criteria are met but another possible cause of dementia is present but judged not to be the main factor, for example, mild vitamin B_{12} deficiency. In centres routinely involved in dementia assessment, these two clinical diagnoses have been found to be about 90 per cent accurate.[17]

In most cases, the definitive assessment process may take two or three visits to be completed, though this can often be shortened if the local doctor has completed the essential investigations before referral to the specialist. Sometimes symptoms are so mild that a firm diagnosis cannot be made and ongoing review over the following 6 to 12 months is arranged.

When dementia is confirmed and the type of dementia identified through the history, examination and investigations, the next question is: should the person with dementia be told the diagnosis? The handling of this issue has changed considerably over time. Twenty years ago, standard practice would have been to only tell the family, unless the person with dementia asked to be told what was wrong or had such a mild disorder that it would be difficult to avoid telling them. Even in these circumstances, full disclosure of the diagnosis would have been the exception rather than the rule.

Now standard practice is to ascertain how much the person with dementia wants to know about what is wrong. In my experience the majority want to be told the diagnosis, although in some cultures this is not the case. The wish to be told the truth comes about partly because we are seeing more people with milder dementias, and partly because of changed community knowledge and attitudes towards health care. There are a number of good reasons for disclosing the diagnosis. It allows the person with dementia to be involved in planning for their future by preparing wills, arranging an enduring power of attorney and possibly enduring guardianship. It gives them the opportunity to utilise their remaining years of relatively intact cognition in the way that they choose. Of course, it also allows the person with dementia to participate actively in treatment planning and, if interested, to participate in dementia support groups. The Alzheimer's Association, which also notes that in more advanced dementia the disclosure of the diagnosis may be neither warranted nor meaningful, supports this general approach.

Giving the diagnosis must be done sensitively, allowing time for the person with dementia to assimilate the information. I usually introduce

the topic bit by bit, initially by describing the abnormalities found; if the person with dementia appears to be becoming distressed, I curtail the extent of information I provide. Often it is the family members who have greatest difficulty with this process. Some would rather that their relative not be told, for fear of the adverse effect knowing the diagnosis may have. In my experience, adverse reactions are quite uncommon, though occasionally some people become depressed. For some others it may be devastating news that they just cannot tolerate, particularly in younger people. In such circumstances, clinicians and families need to be aware that there is a slightly increased risk of suicide in the three months after diagnosis and put extra supports in place if it seems that the person with dementia is not coping with the bad news. However, the initial reaction is often one of relief that there is an explanation for what has been happening to them.[18]

> Eighty-year-old Virginia had been aware that there was something wrong with her memory for some months, though her daughter Penny had been concerned for over a year. The memory clinic had been a daunting experience, and although Virginia couldn't quite remember the precise difficulties that she had with the tests, she knew she had been a little embarrassed about being unable to do them all. Virginia had liked to think that her memory problems were due to her age, but now she was not so sure. When the clinic doctor asked her if she wanted to know what was wrong, she immediately replied 'Of course'. After some explanation of what the tests had shown, she was told that her memory problems were due to Alzheimer's disease. When asked if she understood what that condition was she recalled that Ronald Reagan had been diagnosed with it but did not know much else. Penny obviously knew a bit more, for she looked rather wan.

It is often the children of the person with dementia who express the most concerns at this point. These include the prospects for treatments that might help, fears about their own prospects of developing a dementia and worries about how their aged parent(s) will cope. The spouse of the person with dementia may hold similar concerns, but is often not as vocal. It is critical to provide the family with sufficient information, without overloading them, to allow them to assist in short-term decision-making, for example on treatment options. Health department, pharmaceutical company and Alzheimer's Association brochures about aspects of dementia and its treatment should be provided to the family to read in their own time. I usually direct the family to the Alzheimer's Association website where numerous help sheets can be downloaded (see Appendices 1 and 2).

Initial management

It is impossible to separate dementia assessment from initial management, so I will briefly canvass that topic here. Initial medical management should include cognitive enhancing drugs if the diagnosis is Alzheimer's disease and/or dementia with Lewy bodies and other clinical criteria are met (see Chapter 7). If there are significant behavioural or psychological complications of the dementia such as depression, hallucinations or aggression, various psychotropic drugs could be used (see Chapter 7) or psychosocial treatments recommended (see Chapter 8).

Aside from these treatments, the person with dementia and their family should be encouraged to plan for the future by making sure that they have a valid will, enduring power of attorney and possibly enduring guardianship in place. If they are still driving, a driving assessment, preferably with an occupational therapist, should be recommended to determine competence to drive (see Chapter 12). In some jurisdictions there is mandatory reporting to licensing authorities of persons with dementia who are still driving. Community support services might be required for the more severely affected, particularly if they live alone and need to take medication.

It is also important to recognise that dementia is a chronic disorder that requires long-term commitment of specialist services that are able to interface with local doctors and community services. Follow-up arrangements to monitor progress are recommended. Family caregivers and the person with dementia often require support after the diagnosis, either through the social worker on the specialist team or the Alzheimer's Association.

Summary

The assessment of dementia ranges from initial detection of cognitive change to the full medical, psychological and social evaluation required to make an accurate diagnosis, address any active psychosocial problems, educate the family and commence appropriate treatments. This process is often enhanced by the involvement of a multidisciplinary team.

CHAPTER 7

Drug Treatments

The last decade has seen a mix of advances and retreats in the drug treatments of dementia. What has been achieved so far is merely the tip of the iceberg; much more research will be needed before a cure for any of the dementias can be proclaimed. Current treatments are aimed at ameliorating the symptoms of dementia rather than targeting the underlying causes. Except for a few treatments for specific disorders, current available drug treatments are used in most types of dementia. Here I will consider the main domains of treatment and discuss the different options in each domain. As it is not my intent to provide a 'how to' guide in the management of dementia, I give a broad overview of the different drug types rather than providing a great deal of detail on how to use specific drugs.

Some general principles

All drugs have side effects of some sort; in people with dementia increased confusion is common. As the number of drugs prescribed to an individual increases, the risk of confusion increases. Drugs that are used in the treatment of dementia may take many weeks to show a positive effect, so providing there are no obvious side effects, it is important to give each treatment an adequate trial. However, where a drug causes significant side effects before a positive effect can be determined, it is probably best to discontinue it. In making such a decision, the potential and often intangible long-term benefits need to be considered, so the decision is not always easy.

Memory and cognition: the cognitive (memory) enhancing drugs

As memory impairment is the central disturbance of most dementias, for many people sustained reversal of the memory disorder is seen as being the hallmark of successful treatment. Currently available treatments have been developed for Alzheimer's disease with some limited use in other dementias; therefore regulatory authorities worldwide have, in the most part, only approved them for use in Alzheimer's disease. At present there are no drugs that have been approved for use in frontotemporal dementia or vascular dementia with the exception of when these disorders are co-morbid with Alzheimer's disease. Many drugs used to treat symptoms of dementia are prescribed 'off label'.

With the knowledge that acetycholine is critical to memory function and other cognitions, and that acetylcholine is deficient in Alzheimer's disease, efforts to rectify the deficit have been the focus of much pharmaceutical company research over the last 30 years. Attempts to increase the production of acetylcholine in the brain were largely unsuccessful, in part because most drugs were intolerable. It was only when efforts switched to preserving the acetylcholine still present in the brain that progress was made.

Cholinesterase inhibitors

Drugs of the type known as cholinesterase inhibitors have been the only ones to receive approval for the treatment of mild to moderate Alzheimer's disease. An important issue to note is that, with one exception, these drugs have received approval only for the treatment of Alzheimer's disease, not any other form of dementia. This is because when the evidence was put to regulatory bodies, such as the Food and Drug Administration (FDA) in the US, the National Institute for Health and Clinical Excellence in the UK, and the Therapeutic Goods Administration (TGA) in Australia, all of the major research trials had only involved people with Alzheimer's disease. Later, when new research was put to it, the FDA gave approval for the use of the cholinesterase inhibitor rivastigmine in the treatment of Parkinson's dementia. Research has also demonstrated some benefit in the treatment of dementia with Lewy bodies and vascular dementia but the cholinesterase inhibitors are not approved for use in these conditions because the evidence is not strong enough.[1, 2, 3]

Cholinesterase inhibitors slow the breakdown of acetylcholine in the nerve synapse, thus increasing the amount available for communication

between nerve cells. The first drug to receive marketing approval in the US and Australia was tacrine (Cognex), which was released in Australia in 1993 but is no longer available. Its release was somewhat controversial, as it had very high rates of side effects, mainly gastrointestinal disturbances and liver toxicity that limited its use to the extent that relatively few people were able to tolerate a dose sufficient to obtain much benefit. Those able to tolerate it at the highest strength (around one third of patients) had about 50 per cent chance of obtaining significant improvement of memory function for around a year.

The second drug released was donepezil (Aricept) in 1996 in the US (1997 in Australia and the UK). It has numerous advantages over tacrine including relatively low rates of side effects and once daily dosing as compared with the four times a day regime of tacrine. Donepezil has subsequently become the best-selling Alzheimer's disease treatment despite the release of two other agents, rivastigmine (Exelon) in 1997 in the US (2000 in Australia) and galantamine (Reminyl) in 2001. It should be noted that there is no good evidence that there is any significant difference in the effectiveness of these three drugs.[4, 5] The pharmaceutical companies responsible for each of these drugs have made various efforts to gain market advantage. The tolerability of rivastigmine was improved when the transdermal Exelon patch was released in 2007, while the extended release formulation of galantamine allowing once daily dosing also proved more acceptable to consumers. More recently, a 23mg donepezil tablet was controversially approved by the FDA in 2010 for moderate to severe Alzheimer's disease only months before the patent expired. Concerns have been raised about the dose of the tablet (note that it cannot be achieved using a combination of existing tablet strengths), the tolerability of the high dose, and whether the evidence upon which the decision was made was adequate.[6]

Table 7.1 Cognitive enhancing drugs

	Donepezil	Rivastigmine		Galantamine	Memantine
Drug type	Cholinesterase inhibitor	Cholinesterase inhibitor		Cholinesterase inhibitor	NMDA receptor antagonist
Indication	Mild–severe Alzheimer's disease	Mild–moderate Alzheimer's disease		Mild–moderate Alzheimer's disease	Moderate–severe Alzheimer's disease
Effective daily dose range	5, 10, 23mg tablets	6–12mg capsules	9–18mg patch	16–24mg extended release capsules/tablets (start on 8mg)/oral solution	20mg daily tablets/drops
Dosing regime	Once daily (evening)	Twice daily	Once daily	Once daily (morning)	Once daily
Types of side effects	Nausea, vomiting, diarrhoea, fatigue, dizziness, vivid dreams, slow heart rate, seizures, bladder neck obstruction	Nausea, vomiting, diarrhoea, fatigue, dizziness, headaches, slow heart rate, seizures, bladder neck obstruction		Nausea, vomiting, diarrhoea, anorexia, weight loss, fatigue, somnolence, agitation, slow heart rate, seizures, bladder neck obstruction, tremor	Hallucinations, confusion, headaches, dizziness, gastrointestinal upsets
Tolerability	Well tolerated up to 10mg per day but side effects may outweigh benefits at 23mg	Patch well tolerated, capsules – few able to tolerate the most effective dose of 12mg daily		Well tolerated up to 16mg per day but side effects may outweigh benefits at 24mg	Very well tolerated

Source: American Journal of Psychiatry and NICE [7, 8]

So, how well do the cholinesterase inhibitors work? Put simply, about one third of Alzheimer patients will have a temporary improvement for approximately 12 to 18 months, one third will stabilise for about the same time and the rest will obtain little if any benefit. Some people may benefit for three or more years but it is unclear how often this might happen. There are no established predictors as to which people might benefit although evidence of improvement in the first few weeks is a good sign. An important issue with these drugs is that benefits are only maintained so long as the person keeps taking them. Within a fortnight of cessation, a person who has shown improvement will decline to the presumed level of function that would have occurred without treatment. Thus it is critical that the drugs are taken reliably, as too many missed doses are likely to negate any benefit.

As Table 7.1 shows, gastrointestinal side effects are the most common side effects reported, and tend to be the main reason that drugs are not tolerated. However, with their use in older, frailer patients than were involved as subjects in the drug trial research that originally demonstrated the effectiveness of these drugs, it has become apparent that cardiac problems, including slow heart rate and syncopal episodes, are more common than were previously appreciated. An electrocardiogram is now recommended before starting therapy to ensure that there are no conditions that predispose to those adverse events. Generally speaking, therapeutic doses of donepezil, galantamine and the rivastigmine patch are well tolerated; this is not as often the case with rivastigmine capsules or with high-dose galantamine and donepezil.[9, 10]

What do we mean by improvement? Signs of improvement generally emerge within two or three months though evidence of stabilisation may require at least 12 months of observation. Symptomatic improvement may occur in a number of domains but the most frequently reported areas are better concentration and alertness, improved short-term memory, better global function, improved functional capacity and improved behaviour. This may translate to fewer burdens on family caregivers. Not all people will benefit in all domains; some are more alert and show a greater interest in activities but do not appear to have any changes in memory. Others have memory improvements but do not seem to benefit in other ways. How long benefits may last is unpredictable.

This variability in types of treatment responses is of great importance in countries where regulatory bodies have placed restrictions on their initial and ongoing prescription. In the UK, the National Institute for Health and Clinical Excellence (NICE) guidance recommends initiation

of treatment by a specialist, regular review and continuation only if there is worthwhile effect.[11] In British Columbia, Canada, the drugs are covered under the Alzheimer's Drug Therapy Initiative and can be prescribed by general practitioners. A baseline standardised Mini Mental State Examination (MMSE) score of 10–26 and a Global Deterioration Scale stage four, five or six are required for initial six-month prescription. Thereafter six-monthly reviews are required to determine that the patient remains within these criteria and demonstrates improvement or stability in the previous six months.[12]

Quite reasonably, the intent is to restrict the use of these drugs to people who demonstrate a treatment response. In Australia, until recently, response was defined almost exclusively by cognitive performance, but now improvements in global function or behaviour can be taken into account. As Alzheimer's disease is progressive and on average results in a two or three-point reduction on the MMSE every year, a lack of decline over a year should be regarded as a treatment response.

While there must be a diagnosis of Alzheimer's disease, it should be noted that if there are good clinical grounds to believe that Alzheimer's disease is co-morbid with another type of dementia, the drugs may be prescribed. As it is highly likely that there is co-morbid Alzheimer's disease in most cases of dementia with Lewy bodies and in cases of vascular dementia where there has been gradual progression, most of these patients thus qualify for a trial.

Most people who respond to cholinesterase inhibitors have either responded after three months or are showing promising signs of response though some may take the full six months allowed. Around 50 to 60 per cent of the patients I treat stabilise or improve in the first six months. Other clinicians have anecdotally reported similar results. The availability of three cholinesterase inhibitors means that initial non-responders may obtain a second and sometimes a third treatment trial with one of the alternative drugs.

For how long should these drugs be taken? Basically, cholinesterase inhibitors should be maintained for as long as the perceived benefit outweighs any side effects. A recently published trial from the UK demonstrated the benefits from continuing on donepezil.[13] There will be an inevitable decline in function for all patients eventually, but this in itself is not a reason to stop medication. If the person is declining rapidly over six months (and other causes for the deterioration are excluded), it may be worth considering a trial on a higher dose of the drug. This is easier with

galantamine and donepezil because they are licensed for higher doses. On the higher doses, side effects are often the limiting factor.

Another approach is to trial one of the alternative cholinesterase inhibitors. This approach is controversial, with dementia experts split on its value. I have had some success with it. Others suggest a trial discontinuation of therapy. If no worsening is noted after a fortnight then it means the drug has lost its effect; if the person becomes more confused, less functional or more behaviourally disturbed, this provides evidence that the drug is working and it should be immediately recommenced. Most clinicians wait until the person has been placed into a nursing home before making any changes. It is advisable to wait for three months after placement and then do the trial discontinuation. There is evidence that cholinesterase inhibitors are beneficial in severe Alzheimer's disease too, and in the US donepezil is now licensed for this indication.

Memantine

Memantine has neuroprotective properties and has been approved for use in the treatment of dementia in Germany for over ten years. It appears to have its greatest effect later in the disease process. In Australia, memantine is approved for use in moderately severe Alzheimer's disease.[14] In the UK, the NICE guidance recommends memantine as an option in moderate Alzheimer's disease when patients are intolerant of or have a contraindication to cholinesterase inhibitors or have severe Alzheimer's disease.[15] Memantine appears to protect the brain's nerve cells against glutamate, a neurotransmitter released in excess amounts by cells damaged by Alzheimer's disease and other neurological disorders. Memantine is very well tolerated and can be combined with cholinesterase inhibitors.[16] There is modest evidence that in moderate to severe Alzheimer's disease, combination cholinesterase inhibitor and memantine therapy is more effective than either drug alone,[17] but thus far regulatory authorities around the world have not been sufficiently impressed with the evidence to support the use of two cognitive enhancers simultaneously.

Some unproven cognitive (memory) enhancing drugs
Souvenaid

Souvenaid is a nutritional supplement developed by researchers at the Massachusetts Institute of Technology for persons with prodromal or early Alzheimer's disease. The product, which is taken in a strawberry- or

vanilla-flavoured drink, contains nutrients thought to improve synapse formation (such as omega-3 polyunsaturated fats, phospholipids) along with other nutrients thought to improve memory (such as vitamins E, C, B_6, B_{12} and folic acid).[18] In essence it is a cocktail of many of the vitamins and nutrients discussed in Chapter 2. There are trials that have shown some limited benefit but it is unclear whether this product offers anything more than a balanced diet.[19]

Ginkgo biloba

As described in Chapter 3, the Chinese herb *ginkgo biloba* is thought to increase circulation to the brain. It is prescribed routinely in Europe for memory problems. In Germany ginkgo extracts (240mg a day) have been approved to treat Alzheimer's disease. However, the evidence to support its use is limited with better-quality studies failing to demonstrate efficacy.[20] Although ginkgo does not appear to cause many side effects, it might cause gastric bleeding especially when taken with aspirin. I do not currently recommend the use of ginkgo to my patients.

Vitamin E

There is some modest evidence that vitamin E may slow down the progression of Alzheimer's disease as defined by institutionalisation, functional decline or death. It is unlikely to improve cognition. Although the dose used in the trial that was reported to be effective was 1000 International Units (IU) twice per day, most clinicians recommend 400 IU per day, as there are concerns it can promote bleeding in people with vitamin K deficiency and that doses above that are linked to increased mortality. Though often recommended to be taken in combination with a cognitive enhancing drug, studies have failed to demonstrate additional benefit.[21] I do not recommend the use of vitamin E.

Selegiline

This drug is used in the treatment of Parkinson's disease. There is modest evidence from a number of studies that it can have beneficial effects on memory, mood and behaviour in Alzheimer's disease but insufficient to recommend it in routine clinical use.[22]

Propentofylline

Propentofylline is regarded as a neuroprotective agent because it inhibits the activation of glial cells, which have a role in causing brain

cell destruction. There is limited evidence of modest efficacy in both Alzheimer's disease and vascular dementia. Although it potentially could be used in combination with the cholinesterase inhibitors, propentofylline is not recommended for use in the treatment of dementia in humans and seems to be mainly used in treating lethargic older dogs.

Huperzine A

This is a moss extract that has been used in traditional Chinese medicine for centuries. It has properties similar to the cholinesterase inhibitor drugs and recent Phase II clinical trials have shown potency similar to the established cholinesterase inhibitors. The main problem that delayed the development of huperzine A was lack of uniform standards of manufacture, due to its being regarded as a dietary supplement, and this may result in variation in strength from one batch to the next. Huperzine A should not be used in combination with other approved cholinesterase inhibitors as there is the potential for adverse drug–drug interactions. Two recent reviews published by the Cochrane Collaboration concluded that there is insufficient evidence to support the use of huperzine A in the treatment of Alzheimer's disease and vascular dementia.[23, 24]

Brahmi

This is an Indian Ayurvedic herb popular in India and Japan as a nerve tonic for treating insomnia and nervous tension, and for improving memory. There is no good evidence that it is of any benefit in the treatment or prevention of dementia.

GH3 (Gerovital)

This procaine-based agent, also known as KH3, is heavily promoted as an 'anti-ageing nutrient' which, amongst many claims, may assist 'failing memory' and 'senility'. There is no good evidence that it is of any benefit in the treatment or prevention of dementia, though some people report that they feel less depressed.

Phosphatidylserine

This is a type of fat found in cell membranes and it is supposed to protect cells from damage by bolstering the cell membrane. As this was derived from the brain cells of cows, the outbreak of 'mad cow disease' effectively ended investigations, although early clinical trials showed some interesting results.[25]

Hydergine

Hydergine is a mixture of ergoloid mesylates that has been marketed for the treatment of non-specific cognitive impairment for over 40 years. There have been over 150 clinical trials, some of which have shown some benefit but not to the extent that warrants use in routine clinical practice.[26]

Tramiprosate

Tramiprosate inhibits the formation of amyloid plaque. It was unsuccessfully trialled in a large Phase III clinical study before the sponsor decided to abandon its intention to market it as a prescription drug and instead has been selling it over the internet as a 'medicine food'.[27, 28]

Drugs for the behavioural and psychological symptoms of dementia (BPSD)

Behavioural changes such as agitation, aggression, sexual disinhibition and disruptive vocalisations along with psychological symptoms such as depression, anxiety, paranoid delusions and hallucinations, are often the most distressing part of the process of dementia for both caregivers and the person with dementia. The International Psychogeriatric Association has coined the umbrella term 'behavioural and psychological symptoms of dementia' (BPSD) to describe these clinical features.[29] Other terms that have been used include 'problem behaviours', 'disruptive behaviours', neuropsychiatric symptoms and 'challenging behaviour', the last of these being preferable as it suggests that most behaviours involve an interaction between the caregiver and the person with dementia. I prefer the term 'BPSD' as it also includes the psychological component. BPSD has been found to be the major factor contributing to stress in family and professional caregivers and to the person with dementia being placed into institutional care. In essence, the caregiver gets burnt out from dealing with the behaviour.

Many different psychotropic drugs (drugs used to treat psychiatric disorders) have been used with varying degrees of success to treat these problems. In fact one of the major issues that has arisen worldwide, particularly in nursing homes, is the overuse and misuse of these drugs. In research that I undertook with Henry Brodaty in 1996–97 in 11 Sydney nursing homes, we found that 59 per cent of residents (most of whom had dementia) had been prescribed at least one psychotropic drug in the previous month, and 22 per cent had been prescribed two or more.

About 30 per cent were prescribed sleeping tablets, 25 per cent antipsychotic drugs and 20 per cent antidepressants. Importantly, we found that those prescribed antidepressants had the highest rates of depression and those prescribed antipsychotics the highest rates of psychosis. It appeared that the correct types of drugs were being prescribed but that their effectiveness was questionable.[30]

This raises the fundamental issue about BPSD – the best form of treatment is prevention. Although changes in brain function underpin BPSD, often the extent to which behaviour becomes a challenge is determined by the way in which caregivers interact with the person with dementia and the appropriateness of the environmental milieu. For example, BPSD is more likely to occur in a noisy environment with caregivers who do not take the time to communicate clearly. This is covered in more detail in Chapter 8. There is also evidence that cholinesterase inhibitors reduce the emergence of BPSD in Alzheimer's disease, although there is little evidence that they are effective in reducing existing behaviour except in patients with psychosis associated with dementia with Lewy bodies where they seem to be reasonably effective.[31]

It is also important to realise that just because a person with dementia has a certain behaviour or psychological symptom, this does not automatically mean that it should be treated. Unless BPSD is distressing the person with dementia or causing significant problems for others around the person with dementia, it may be best left as it is. If treatment is required, non-drug (psychosocial) treatments should always be considered first. Pharmacotherapy of behavioural changes should be reserved for severe disturbances where adequate trials of psychosocial treatments have failed or the urgency of the situation requires an immediate intervention. Another circumstance where psychotropic drugs should be used is where the person with dementia has a pre-existing psychiatric disorder such as depression, bipolar disorder or schizophrenia, requiring maintenance therapy for the person to remain well. Even if drugs are used, psychosocial treatments will usually be needed in combination with them. All drugs should be prescribed at the lowest effective dose. I will consider psychosocial treatments in Chapter 8.

Another important issue is consent for treatment. The broader issue of mental competence and the determination of capacity is considered in Chapter 12. As the majority of people with dementia prescribed psychotropics for BPSD will have lost their capacity to consent, it is essential that legal consent be obtained. The precise process varies from

jurisdiction to jurisdiction around the world. In the state of New South Wales, Australia, psychotropic drugs are classified as a 'major medical treatment' and as such require *written consent* from the legally defined 'person responsible' – usually the spouse, child, sibling or legal guardian of the person. Some years ago we audited the files from three Sydney nursing homes and found that in only 6.5 per cent of persons without capacity to consent were all of the consent regulations adhered to by the doctor when psychotropic medication was prescribed. It was unclear in how many other cases verbal consent had been obtained. This lack of legal consent is an issue of great concern.[32]

A third issue is the use of drugs as a form of chemical restraint – in other words, where psychotropic drugs are used simply to sedate the person with dementia rather than being used for their therapeutic effects. Usually this involves excessive dosing, with the person with dementia left in an oversedated, drowsy state for most of the time. While this might occur inadvertently during efforts to control severe agitation and aggression, it should only be a transient phase as the correct dose of medication is sought. Chronic oversedation is dangerous, inappropriate, unnecessary and unethical.

Here I will consider some of the more commonly prescribed psychotropic drugs along with the main indications for their use (summarised in Table 7.2).

Table 7.2 Drugs for the behavioural and psychological symptoms of dementia

Type	Examples
Atypical antipsychotics	Risperidone, olanzapine, quetiapine
Other antipsychotics	Haloperidol, trifluoperazine
SSRI antidepressants	Sertraline, citalopram, paroxetine, fluvoxamine, escitalopram
Other antidepressants	Venlafaxine, mirtazepine, moclobemide, duloxetine, trazodone
Mood stabilisers	Carbamazepine, sodium valproate
Benzodiazepines	Oxazepam, temazepam, lorazepam

cont.

Type	Examples
Other sedatives	Zopiclone, melatonin
Hormonal treatments	Cyproterone acetate
Analgesics	Paracetamol, codeine, morphine, buprenorphine patch

Antipsychotic drugs

Antipsychotics are primarily designed to treat psychoses such as schizophrenia. For many years they have also been used in the management of dementia. As one might expect, psychotic symptoms such as suspiciousness, false beliefs (delusions), accusations, paranoia, and hallucinations have been a target, but they are perhaps more frequently used for treating aggressive behaviours, agitation and sexual disinhibition.

Only in the past decade have a few good studies to determine their effectiveness been completed. These studies have yielded mixed results and there has also been controversy related to the safe use of both the atypical antipsychotic drugs such as risperidone, olanzapine and quetiapine as well as the older antipsychotics such as haloperidol. This means that they should be used with caution and in general only after trials of psychosocial treatments have failed.[33, 34] Basically there is now evidence that these drugs may significantly increase the risk of cerebrovascular events such as stroke by up to threefold, as well as mortality, in persons with dementia. This has resulted in a statement by the UK Committee on the Safety of Medicines[35] and an advisory note from the US Food and Drug Administration regarding the use of antipsychotics in dementia.[36]

In addition a US National Institute of Mental Health sponsored study (CATIE-AD) compared the effectiveness of risperidone, quetiapine and olanzapine with placebo in treating aggression, agitation or psychosis using the pragmatic outcome measure of 'discontinuation due to any reason' and found no significant benefit to any of the drugs. While olanzapine and risperidone appeared to be efficacious compared with placebo, adverse effects offset these benefits. It was concluded that use of atypical antipsychotics should be restricted to patients who have few or no adverse effects and for whom benefits can be discerned.[37]

The general advantage of the atypical antipsychotics over the older antipsychotics is their lower rate of side effects. For example, parkinsonian side effects – shuffling gait, stooped posture, slowed movements and

increased risk of falls – occur in only 2 to 5 per cent of recipients compared with around 20 per cent who develop these side effects with haloperidol. Other problems include confusion, sedation and constipation. Risperidone is the only oral atypical antipsychotic approved for use in dementia in Australia, largely because it has the best evidence of efficacy even though it is only modest. The starting dose is 0.5mg per day with the maximum dose of 2mg per day.[38] No antipsychotics have FDA approval in the treatment of dementia in the US.

Of the older antipsychotics, haloperidol (0.5–1.5mg) has the best evidence of efficacy. After a few months use, however, there is a higher risk of developing tardive dyskinesia, which involves involuntary movements, in particular with the mouth and tongue. It is quite distressing and unsightly and it is often permanent.[39]

Antipsychotic drugs are best avoided in dementia with Lewy bodies (DLB) due to their propensity to cause severe parkinsonism in this condition at very low dosage. As hallucinations are common in DLB, treatments are often required but fortunately the cholinesterase inhibitor drugs seem to be effective in settling such psychotic symptoms. If this is ineffective, a low dose of quetiapine (25–50mg) might be tolerated.

> Roger had always had a short temper but now he seemed to strike out at the least provocation. He seemed suspicious of others and had made no close friends in the nursing home. The nursing staff treated him gingerly as he had hit them a few times. Eventually, after numerous efforts to manage him without drugs, a trial of risperidone was commenced. After some weeks Roger was obviously less suspicious and less irritable. Aggressive outbursts were now containable through diversional strategies.

How long should these drugs be prescribed? If the target behaviours or symptoms have remained under control for three months then I recommend a trial discontinuation. There is evidence that the longer the drugs are prescribed, the greater the risk of adverse effects including higher mortality.[40] One of the major problems in nursing homes is the failure to have trial discontinuations of these drugs after three months treatment.

Antidepressant drugs
Antidepressant drugs are mainly used to treat depression and anxiety, but can be used for disruptive vocalisations, agitation and sleep disturbances. Their effectiveness in treating depression and anxiety associated with dementia is limited with two large studies in the US and the UK showing

no benefit over placebo, though some good individual results are obtained.[41, 42] One reason for the limited effectiveness is that depression associated with dementia does not always have typical features, so that accurate diagnosis is harder.[43] Another is that the brain damage caused by the dementia inhibits the action of the drugs.

There are many different classes of antidepressants but in general, there are the older drugs, such as the tricyclic antidepressants, and the newer drugs, particularly the selective serotonin reuptake inhibitors (SSRIs). As with the antipsychotic drugs, the main difference between the older and newer drugs is the higher rate of side effects with the older drugs; there is little difference in the effectiveness of individual antidepressants. Possibly the older drugs work better with very severe depression.

Experts consistently recommend the SSRI antidepressants as the first-line treatment of depression and anxiety in older people, whether or not these conditions are associated with dementia. The drug of choice is usually citalopram (10–30mg per day) as it has been shown to be effective in depression associated with dementia and has the lowest risk of drug interactions.[44] All SSRIs can have side effects that include nausea, vomiting, diarrhoea, agitation and falls. There is also a risk of sodium depletion, which may cause confusion, lethargy and weakness, so the person's sodium levels need to be checked. If SSRIs are ineffective, then the main treatment options are probably venlafaxine, trazodone or moclobemide. Antidepressants should generally be prescribed for a minimum of six months if they are effective.

Mood-stabilising drugs

These drugs are used to treat epilepsy, chronic pain and bipolar (manic-depressive) illness. The main indications for their use in dementia are aggression, agitation and mood instability. There is only limited evidence for their effectiveness, but carbamazepine or sodium valproate can be useful with aggressive behaviour if other treatments have failed. Side effects are largely related to sedation, unsteady gait and liver dysfunction. They tend to be dose related and serum levels are available to assist in finding the optimal dose.[45]

Sedative-hypnotic and anxiolytic drugs

Most of these drugs are in the benzodiazepine class and they are of very limited use in dementia, as they tend to oversedate.[46] There is also the possibility of a paradoxical reaction in which agitation worsens instead of

abating. They can be useful in settling acute anxiety reactions if limited to a few doses. Night sedation is the main indication in circumstances where non-drug treatments have been ineffective, and here the short-acting temazepam is the first choice as it is less likely to cause a hangover effect in the morning. However, melatonin is the drug of choice for sleep disturbances as it has few side effects.

Antiandrogens

These are used in men with recalcitrant sexually inappropriate behaviour and/or aggression. The main drug is cyproterone acetate, which works by suppressing testosterone levels. This is a controversial treatment and regarded as second or third-line option after other treatment trials have failed. In New South Wales, Australia, the Guardianship Tribunal has to provide consent for this treatment for a mentally incompetent person even when there is a legal guardian in place. I have prescribed it several times with success.

Analgesics

I mention analgesics (painkillers) here because pain is a common factor in BPSD and is notoriously poorly treated in older people. A recent randomised controlled trial found that a systematic approach to pain management significantly reduced agitation in people with moderate to severe dementia in nursing homes.[47] Analgesics can range from simple treatments such as aspirin and paracetamol through to narcotic analgesics such as morphine and buprenorphine transdermal patch. In advanced dementia where communication is limited, a restless bedbound person may well be in serious discomfort but unable to communicate it verbally other than by screaming or extreme restlessness. Presuming factors such as chronic constipation and other obvious causes of pain have been excluded, a palliative care approach to treatment by using optimal doses of narcotic analgesics to relieve distress without oversedation is sensible.

Mary had been in the nursing home for 18 months with advanced dementia. She no longer spoke intelligibly and was bedbound. To the consternation of staff, residents and neighbours, Mary would scream out in a loud high-pitched voice for many hours every day. No particular reason could be identified for the noise. She called out whether or not family were present, at all times of the day and night, before and after meals, before and after personal care from nurses. Distraction, attention, touch, aromatherapy and music therapy made no difference. Various antipsychotic and

antidepressant drugs had no impact. Simple analgesics were ineffective. Eventually, in desperation, mist morphine was commenced and within days the noise improved, although it never stopped. This was sufficient for staff and residents to obtain some respite.

Medical problems that impact on the dementia

In earlier chapters, I indicated that a range of medical conditions including hypertension, diabetes mellitus, cardiac disorders, high cholesterol, hypothyroidism and vitamin B_{12} and folate deficiency may contribute to cognitive changes. Thus it is important that they be optimally treated to maximise function. This will be particularly important in people with vascular dementia. Drugs commonly required include antihypertensives, antiplatelet drugs (aspirin), diuretics and the replacement of all vitamin and hormone deficiencies.

Epileptic fits may occur later in the course of dementia, where anticonvulsant drugs may be needed. Here sodium valproate or carbamazepine may be the drugs of choice due to their potential benefits on behaviour. Urinary incontinence is often a problem that can make or break community care; if this is the case a trial of low-dose oxybutynin might be considered. As it tends to have the opposite effect to the cholinesterase inhibitors it can increase confusion, and so is a treatment to be used cautiously. Falls are another common problem in people with dementia and these frequently result in hip fractures. Swallowing difficulties increase as dementia progresses and this may result in recurrent bouts of aspiration pneumonia.[48]

Summary

The current drug treatments of dementia symptoms are modestly effective but have significant shortcomings so there is much room for improvement. There are two main areas of treatment – drugs which target cognition and also seem to benefit behaviour and function, and drugs which target the behavioural and psychological symptoms of dementia.

CHAPTER 8

Psychosocial Treatments

Dementia can be such a distressing condition that the importance of continuing to 'live life' is lost to many people. This is a complex topic that has many nuances.

Whole books have been written about how to interact with persons with dementia. In this chapter, rather than writing a condensed version of one of the excellent books that have a practical 'how to' focus (see list in Appendix 3), I outline common psychosocial approaches that are utilised in dementia care, most of which are based upon the attainment of wellbeing. The themes that emerge will, it is hoped, provide some guidance about living with dementia.

Person-centred care

Tom Kitwood in the UK drew attention to the importance of personhood in dementia. He based his approach on the assumption that humans have five basic psychological needs – comfort, attachment, inclusion, occupation and identity – that in themselves gather around the central need for love.[1] To understand these needs in the individual it is important to know the person's biography and personality so that their perspective of the situation can be respectfully integrated into their care and their opinions valued.

It has become increasingly recognised that person-centred approaches to care underpin many effective interventions. Although person-centred care is a term describing an approach used by health professionals to meet the needs of their patients, for persons with dementia it also applies to their interactions with family and caregivers. In health care settings, person-centred care, in which the individual's needs and preferences are considered from a holistic perspective, is contrasted with task-centred

care in which the focus is upon a specific task, such as dressing a wound or giving out medication. A similar contrast can be made to approaches used by family caregivers. Dementia Care Mapping was developed out of person-centred care by the Bradford Group in the UK and it is both an evaluative instrument and vehicle for applying person-centred dementia care. A recent randomised controlled trial showed no advantage of this approach over standard person-centred care, but the implementation costs of the latter were less than 25 per cent of those for Dementia Care Mapping due to the intensive staff training required.[2]

Person-centred care also resonates with the increasing empowerment of people with early dementia that has been manifested through activities such as disclosure of diagnosis and involvement in their own care planning as well as through their participation in community consultations about dementia care, support groups for people with dementia, and giving presentations at dementia conferences. Some of the most powerful conference presentations that I have witnessed in recent years were by persons with mild dementia, with themes such as fighting the stigma of dementia and the importance of having meaningful activities to live with a good quality of life in dementia.

Some general rules of communication

There are some general rules about communication with a person with dementia that are worth mentioning. Remember that the person is dementing, not demented. This means that many mental functions remain relatively intact until the later stages of illness, and these retained abilities should be tapped *as much as possible*. Another common mistake that caregivers and other people make is to talk down to the person as if they are a child or not present at all. Such an approach is both demeaning and likely to provoke resentment. Try to communicate on an adult-to-adult level but keep things simple. Short sentences containing only one subject are better than longer ones. When asking questions, avoid the 'multiple choice' approach. For example, rather than asking 'Would you like to go to the movies, go to the concert or out to a restaurant?', it would be better to break down the question into two parts. Use gestures, speak slowly and clearly but try not to be stilted. Communication should also be tailored to the needs of each person by respecting them as a unique individual who had a life before their illness (as well as now) and whose feelings need to be recognised and respected. In other words, take a person-centred approach.

Mild dementia

I am not exactly sure how I would react if I was told I had Alzheimer's disease. Maybe I would be like many of my better-informed patients these days, who already suspect the diagnosis and to whom its confirmation comes as no surprise. That doesn't mean that the diagnosis isn't upsetting, but at least it removes uncertainty and provides an opportunity to plan for the future. There are many other types of reactions. It might be depressing, as any bad news would be, but most people want to face it and not avoid it. To some, however, it may be absolutely devastating.[3] Some people acknowledge the diagnosis, then simply forget what they have been told, or go into denial about it. Others just don't want to know, but that reaction is uncommon.

Emotional support and lifestyle advice

Most people want their family, close friends and doctor to be emotionally supportive during this period. Support groups for persons with mild dementia are becoming increasingly common as more people in our ageing population are being diagnosed earlier in the course of their illness. Tom Kitwood, who wrote extensively on this topic, used the term 'holding' as a metaphor for providing a safe place where frightening emotions can be experienced without the person with dementia being overwhelmed by them.[4]

For health care professionals, the technical terms used for emotional support are 'supportive psychotherapy' and 'counselling'. These psychological therapies are simply intended to allow the recipient an opportunity to ventilate their feelings with an attentive, empathic person who is non-judgemental in the support they provide. Some basic advice and information about planning for the future and legal decisions, as described in Chapter 6, may be given as part of the process of assisting the person with dementia in adjusting to their changed circumstances.

One piece of advice that I regularly offer is encouraging the person with dementia and their family to maintain as much of their usual lifestyle for as long as possible. Tom Kitwood used the term 'celebration' to describe the various simple activities that the person with dementia can enjoy with friends and family to maintain life – singing, walking, eating good meals.[5] Some precautions may need to be taken; for example, trips to distant locations may lead to increased confusion so the person with dementia should always travel with an informed caregiver. Yet on the whole, few changes in lifestyle are required for most people with mild dementia.

Memory training (cognitive training/rehabilitation)

People with mild cognitive impairment and mild dementia may benefit from memory training in order to enhance their residual memory function. Probably the most common strategies taught involve the use of 'external memory aids'. Most of us use external memory aids regularly, such as diaries, shopping lists, alarm clocks and message boards in the kitchen. For the person with memory deficits who is not in the habit of using any of these aids, the most difficult thing to achieve is the regular use of the aid. This often requires regular input from a caregiver, as well as from the therapist, to get things going. The use of diaries and message books are probably the most common techniques. Both allow the person with dementia and their caregivers to add items as they arise. Thus a caregiver might write the time they are going to pick up the person with dementia for a shopping trip in the diary, or leave a prominent message on the message board about a forthcoming event. The person with dementia is encouraged to write all day-to-day tasks into their diary, including what people tell them on telephone calls. By habitually referring to their memory aids, they can minimise the impact of short-term memory impairment. Other forms of external memory aids include regular phone calls from a caregiver to remind the person with dementia to take their tablets, automatic pill dispensers with alarms and the use of the alarm clock function on a mobile phone to draw attention to a reminder message on the phone. More complex prospective and retrospective memory aids that are still in development and have yet to be adequately tested in persons with dementia are discussed in Chapter 13. These approaches are suitable in mild to moderate dementia.

New learning can also be enhanced by the appropriate use of cues. Cues are commonly used in study techniques to improve recall for examinations. Students might use lists, acronyms, pictures, visual imagery when they study. A similar approach can be encouraged to counter mild memory deficits due to mild cognitive impairment and dementia. As with study techniques, self-generated cues are more likely to work. The person with dementia is asked to think of questions or images to remind them of what they are learning. Such associations assist later recall of the information. Because it is essential not to overload the person with dementia with trivial information, this approach is best reserved for the items most important to them. It also needs to be done in a manner that is relaxing and not onerous. When efforts to enhance learning resemble being in school, they are bound to fail, especially if the process provokes anxiety.

Another way of enhancing new learning of specific events is to ensure that the event stands out from the daily routine. Having a daily routine for a person with dementia reduces the information load that they have to assimilate, and reduces their stress levels. For an important event such as a birthday party, enrichment of the occasion with the person with dementia's favourite music, colourful decorations, favourite food and close friends will assist the person with dementia to remember the occasion.

Although these memory-training techniques are popular and seem sensible, at present there is very limited evidence of effectiveness in improving memory.[6] Their main role may be to provide structure and routine for persons with dementia and their caregivers. Current Australian studies are examining the effectiveness of computer-based training programmes.[7]

Making memories

One interesting project sponsored by the Alzheimer's Association in Australia a few years ago as a competition, involved persons with early dementia putting together an autobiography that can assist them as the disease progresses. This might involve audio tapes, video tapes, diaries, photos and other bits of nostalgia from their life. The winning entry was an innovative memory quilt. It is unclear whether this approach is beneficial, but some people might find it a lot of fun to do and for those who are interested it seems to me a good idea. There are commercially available DVDs and other products based on digital technology to help this type of project, many of which can be found on the AT Dementia website (see Appendix 2).

Cognitive stimulation therapy

Cognitive stimulation therapy (CST) was developed in the UK and involves an initial 14-session twice-weekly group intervention and a subsequent 24-session weekly maintenance intervention that follows the principles of person-centred care. Each session has themed activities that aim to actively stimulate and engage people with dementia while at the same time providing an optimal learning environment and social interaction. Session themes include games, food, using money, orientation and current affairs. Members name their group and are encouraged to take roles within the group according to their interests and abilities. The aim of the CST programme is to provide an environment for people to learn

and strengthen their existing resources. Reminiscence is integrated within the programme.[8]

It has become a popular approach in the UK largely due to the National Institute for Health and Clinical Excellence (NICE) guidance that recommends its use in mild Alzheimer's disease while placing restrictions upon prescription of cognitive-enhancing drugs to moderate Alzheimer's disease.[9] Evaluations suggest improvements in memory and orientation to a similar level found by cognitive-enhancing drugs. A review included in the 2011 *World Alzheimer Report* concluded that CST had the 'strongest evidence by far' for cognitive benefits.[10] More research is required into CST, particularly regarding the efficacy of individual therapy, longer-term outcomes, and its use in other countries and cultural settings.[11] We are currently running a pilot study of an Australian adaptation.

Moderate to severe dementia

Numerous therapies have been designed to assist in communicating with, stimulating and comforting people with moderate to severe dementia. Some of the therapies overlap and to date there is not much evidence that any particular approach is generally more effective than any other, although individuals might respond better to one approach rather than another. It is most likely that there is a lot of common ground and in part they are likely to work by providing professional and family caregivers with some tools to help them in interacting with the person with dementia. The importance of such assistance should not be underestimated, for coping with a person with dementia can be an overwhelming prospect for the inexperienced. Choice is probably helpful in itself; being able to tap into a variety of different approaches and therapies may be useful.

Routines are an important feature of most therapies – setting aside a period of time each day to do something can assist in structuring the day for both the person with dementia and caregiver alike. Another thing that must be remembered is that most therapies only have an effect in and around the period of their application. Thus a behavioural disturbance might be settled for the duration of the therapy and an hour or two after, but not much longer. It might be necessary to have another therapy session routinely organised for that time, possibly of a different type of therapy, to help quell the re-emerging behaviour.

Validation therapy

Naomi Feil developed validation therapy between 1963 and 1980 to assist in communicating with people who have dementia and other disorders with cognitive impairment. It is a humane practical approach that emphasises stage-specific communication techniques. The principal assumption underlying validation therapy is that all behaviour has meaning, even if the behaviour is extremely inappropriate or based on psychotic experiences. Its main technique is to validate the person with dementia's emotions by acknowledging their feelings, even when they may be based on misinterpretations or misperceptions. The goal of therapy is to make the person with dementia as happy as possible.[12]

> Meg was experiencing hallucinations in which she saw masked intruders come into her room. She worried that they might assault her and thus screamed in distress. The first nurse who came tried to reassure her by telling her that she was just imagining the men and so she wasn't at any risk. Meg remained very scared and kept screaming. A second nurse comforted her by saying 'It must be very scary to have strange men in your room,' which allowed Meg to agree and describe how terrified she had been. Eventually Meg calmed down and seemed more at ease.
>
> The second nurse used a validation therapy approach to communication. By acknowledging Meg's fear, this nurse demonstrated empathy with Meg's plight. The type of reassurance offered by the first nurse had the unintended effect of invalidating Meg's emotions. In reasonably insightful people who experience hallucinations, reassurance that the hallucinations are not real might work providing that acknowledgement of how distressing the hallucinations are accompanies the reassurance.

Feil classifies individuals with cognitive impairment as being at one of four stages on a continuum of dementia. These stages are 'malorientation', 'time confusion', 'repetitive motion' and 'vegetation' and all occur in the previously described moderate and severe stages of dementia. While validation therapy was not designed for mild dementia, the basic technique of validating the person's emotions is derived from counselling psychology and would still be applicable. In general, validation therapy aims to work with the person with dementia's spared abilities and functions while bolstering those that are more severely affected.[13]

Feil describes numerous benefits of validation therapy. These include restoration of the self-worth of the person with dementia, minimisation of the degree to which people with dementia withdraw from the outside world, promotion of communication and interaction with other people,

reduction of stress and anxiety, stimulation of dormant potential, help in resolving unfinished life tasks, and facilitation of independent living for as long as possible. To date, there has been relatively little empirical research to investigate these claims and so the extent to which validation therapy achieves these benefits is unknown. A major problem is that research in this area is very difficult to undertake in a fashion that satisfies most academics that the therapy has a specific benefit and a Cochrane Collaboration review concluded that there was insufficient evidence to allow any conclusion about efficacy.[14] However, qualitative research that has observed validation therapy being used, and anecdotal experience, suggest that there are positive effects especially on the mood of the person with dementia.[15]

There are a number of criticisms of validation therapy. Possibly the most common is that some caregivers find this style of communication very difficult to use because they feel that they are 'colluding' with delusions. Caregivers who must be 'right' or be 'in control' seem to have the most problems, particularly where the relationship with the person with dementia was marked by confrontation before the onset of dementia. Others say that validation therapy is more an attitude towards caregiving rather than a formal therapy. To me, the general approach appears very sensible, non-confrontational and positive.

Reminiscence therapy

Robert Butler in the US first described reminiscence or 'life review' therapy in 1963. It is based on the premise that reminiscence is beneficial for people in the later stages of their life because it provides them with an opportunity to review and reorganise the events of their life in response to the biological and psychological fact of impending death. From this it can be seen that reminiscence therapy is not specifically designed for persons with dementia; indeed, it has been used more frequently to treat depression, to assist in socialisation and as an aid for successful ageing.[16, 17]

In people with dementia, the goals of reminiscence therapy are to decrease isolation and improve morale and wellbeing by triggering memories of past life events. It is usually conducted in a group setting on a weekly basis, often in a day care centre or residential aged care facility. Music and other cues such as photos, videos and books are used to trigger memories. The choice of cues should be relevant to group members, so the group leader will require information on the group members' backgrounds. There is evidence that reminiscence therapy can reduce depressive

symptoms, improve life satisfaction and facilitate communication.[18] Note, however, that some people may not be suited to reminiscence therapy, particularly those who have endured horrific life experiences such as the Holocaust.

It is a technique that can be used in interactions with moderate to severely impaired people with dementia, as a way of stimulating pleasant memories, possibly as a distraction when the person with dementia is upset, or as a way to provide mental stimulation. Some people with mild dementia may use reminiscence techniques as part of a memory training programme, for example, in attempting to remember the names of classmates at school.

> *Percy had been feeling miserable all day and was quite grumpy whenever his wife Norma tried to find out what was wrong. Eventually she decided to play their favourite song 'The Girl from Ipanema' and started talking with Percy about the fun times they had at the Saturday night dances. Percy seemed to brighten with the music and with a little encouragement started dancing with Norma while reminiscing happily about their courtship.*

A Cochrane Collaboration review concluded that although there were promising indications of the effectiveness of reminiscence therapy in dementia, the low quality of published studies prevents any robust conclusions being drawn.[19] Better quality research is required.

Reality orientation

Reality orientation was first described in 1966 as a technique to improve the quality of life of confused older people. It is mainly designed for people with moderate to severe dementia and involves the presentation of orientation and memory information in a group or individual setting in order to provide the person with dementia with a greater understanding of their surroundings and to improve their sense of control and self-esteem. There are two types of reality orientation therapy – continuous and classroom. Continuous 24-hour reality orientation is mainly practised in residential care settings where staff involve the residents with dementia in reality-based communication in every contact throughout the day. Classroom reality orientation is where groups meet on a regular basis to engage in orientation-related activities.[20]

Devices that can be used to assist in the therapy include calendars, clocks, scrapbooks, television and video, educational sessions and newspapers. Typically, there is a noticeboard that displays information

including the weather, day, date, place and forthcoming meals and outings. (Unfortunately, in my experience, many noticeboards are not updated with current information, thus defeating their purpose.) All of these devices are used to stimulate conversation about what is happening in the 'real' world and to assist in practising skills such as grooming, feeding and socialising. It is a reasonably simple technique that can be adapted to many settings.

Critics of reality orientation claim that it is often applied in a mechanistic fashion that is insensitive to the individual needs of the person with dementia, and that the constant relearning of material may contribute to the lowering of self-esteem and mood.[21] In fact, it was such concerns that contributed to Naomi Feil's development of validation therapy and the loss of popularity of the reality orientation technique. However, there is quite good research evidence that reality orientation can have beneficial effects on memory, orientation and behaviour, and this was reflected in a Cochrane Collaboration review that was withdrawn in 2007 because the authors, who were involved in developing cognitive stimulation therapy, felt that the way forward for reality orientation was to incorporate it into cognitive stimulation therapy as described earlier.[22]

Music therapy

Music therapy is more than simply playing music in the background for its calming effects. It is a well-established therapy used in the treatment of a range of mental disorders. Music can evoke emotions that may not be easily tapped into through other means as noted earlier in the chapter in the scenario with Percy. Most of us have experienced the powerful nostalgic reminiscence cued by songs that are associated with particular events in our life – a tune our parents enjoyed, or the one we first danced to with our spouse are common examples. In people who may be having some difficulties in dealing with psychological trauma, music may assist the therapist in helping them talk about it.

For people with dementia, music therapy has two main functions. First, it provides a pleasurable experience through both listening and participation. Regular groups in which the music therapist may play a combination of recorded and live music that allows the participants to listen, sing and play instruments are often a feature of many day care centres and aged care facilities. This type of therapy is largely intended to improve quality of life through social interaction and diversion.

The second function is as a specific therapy designed to reduce behavioural disturbances in aged care facilities. Quiet music played during

mealtimes can reduce agitation and result in greater compliance with eating. Research has shown that when the individual's musical preferences are used in a music therapy programme (as opposed to no music or a standard musical selection), behavioural disturbances are reduced. This may seem self-evident but too often the music played in facilities does not reflect the choices of the residents. I once visited a nursing home to advise on the management of a noisy resident. While I was in her room, the radio was booming with rap music that was clearly being enjoyed by the young cleaner who was there but none of the older residents. (If I had to listen to rap music all day I think that I would get quite noisy!)

An evidence-based review of psychosocial treatments of behavioural symptoms in dementia concluded that preferred music was an effective treatment for agitated and aggressive behaviour though the effect was moderate.[23]

Physical exercise and activity programmes

In Chapter 2, I discussed the potential role of physical exercise in the prevention of dementia. It should come as no surprise that exercise can also be beneficial for persons with dementia. For the person who has been very physically active through their life, it is important to maintain that activity. Often participation in sports such as golf and lawn bowls wanes as the dementia progresses due to declining skills, loss of initiative and family concerns about safety. Dancing and walking are recreational pursuits that can be maintained for much longer if there is a regular partner who can guide the person with dementia. I always encourage participation in a favoured physical activity for as long as possible, even if it requires modification of the person with dementia's involvement. Older persons who withdraw from physical activity due to their health often become unhappy and demoralised, and some become clinically depressed.

Physical exercise is also very useful for people who have not been very active over the years and for those who are in nursing homes. The type of activity may need to be varied to suit the individual; if the person has limited mobility, for example, gentle bending and stretching exercises whilst seated can be beneficial. Whatever type of exercise the person with dementia is encouraged to do, the most important thing is that it is enjoyable. Group games with a ball, musical games, dances, walks, aerobics, resistance training – the list is almost endless. The exercise should also be undertaken regularly, at least 30 minutes per day five times per week. There is good evidence that optimal physical activity can improve sleep

patterns, reduce depressive symptoms and settle behavioural disturbances such as agitation, noisiness and aggression.[24]

Non-exercise-based activity programmes are also important. Singing, art, bingo, television, discussion groups, relaxation therapy, humour therapy and various group games provide mental stimulation to help alleviate boredom and to encourage appropriate social interaction in day care centres and aged care facilities. There is overlap between therapies so discussion groups may involve reminiscence and reality orientation techniques, and so on.

I have regularly advised on the use of selected videotapes based upon the person with dementia's known interests. Anecdotally I have observed that videos of favourite sporting events, concerts and of course old films can be repeatedly shown and have a calming effect if the choice is right for the individual. If the video is not suited to the individual it is usually of little benefit.

Aromatherapy and touch therapy

Most people enjoy a pleasant fragrance and a soothing touch. It is little wonder that aromatherapy and touch therapy, including massage, may have a role in dementia care. Both therapies are forms of complementary medicine and have an extensive history and rationale for their use in various conditions. I don't pretend to understand these therapies at that level; I do regard them as having the potential to improve the person with dementia's quality of life through the provision of pleasant experiences.

Aromatherapy with essential oils has been used mainly as a calming or relaxing influence during the day and as a mild sedative at night. Essential oils are usually applied by room fragrancers, but they can also be delivered in baths, by massage and through inhalations. Lavender oil is possibly the most frequently used oil, particularly for sleep disturbances. Sometimes a lavender bag is placed under the pillow. Other commonly used oils include lemon balm, chamomile, bergamot, sandalwood and rose. There is mounting evidence of good quality that aromatherapy is effective in treating agitation.[25]

We often forget how important it is for us to have direct human contact. Cuddling and holding hands are more than just displays of affection between lovers. There is evidence that such contact increases brain serotonin levels and helps to make us feel happy and content. Similarly, therapeutic massage not only has a direct effect on the muscles being massaged, it also has a general soothing influence on our minds. Many older people in

nursing homes have very little opportunity to get such contact and often crave human touch from visitors. Not surprisingly, studies have shown that both hand massage and therapeutic touch reduce agitated behaviours in nursing home residents. Of course, touch and massage don't need to be as formalised as this but simply incorporated within routine care programmes as a regular part of day-to-day interaction, providing it is acceptable to the person with dementia. A few people prefer not to be touched and this should be respected.

Simulated presence therapy

It is a frequent observation in nursing homes that persons with severe dementia are more content when family members are present. Simulated presence therapy uses audio tapes prepared by family members about past experiences and other personal nostalgia. The families are instructed to talk to the person with dementia and ask questions, leaving gaps so that the person with dementia can answer. Often the person with dementia is observed to respond to the tape as if their family member were present. The same tape can be used repeatedly as at this stage of dementia it is quickly forgotten. There is only limited evidence that it is effective in calming agitated behaviours.[26] However, this therapy has many attractions for me. It is sensible, inexpensive and involves the family at a time many members feel they are unable to contribute much. While I have not seen any reports of using family videos in the same way, this is likely to be another possible application.

Behaviour management

Behaviour management is based on learning theory and is used to eliminate unwanted behaviours and to encourage desirable behaviours in people with moderate to severe dementia. There has been much debate about how much can be learnt at this stage of dementia and for this reason critics of the therapy claim that it is a fundamentally flawed approach. However, several small Australian studies have demonstrated that sufficient learning can occur to allow for the successful treatment of noisy and intrusive behaviours.[27]

The fundamentals of behaviour therapy are familiar to all of us – rewarding desirable behaviours encourages behaviour change. Most parents use variations of this theme in raising their children. The trick is to work out an appropriate reward for the person with dementia that will be sufficient to encourage change. Food, drink and pleasurable activities

are the rewards most frequently used but it may take a while to identify the right reward for the individual.

At the same time, unwanted behaviours should be ignored. The mistake that many people make here is to punish rather than ignore. Punishment definitely should not be a part of a behaviour therapy programme. It may be hard to ignore some types of behaviour and it may be difficult for caregivers to tolerate the behaviour, especially as a behaviour therapy programme needs to be applied consistently for some weeks to be effective. This is often a major limiting factor in the application of behaviour therapy in residential care, as a collaboration of clinical aged care researchers that I led found in a study of the treatment of noisy nursing home residents in Australia. Nursing staff reported that behaviour programmes were often too time consuming to apply when they were already extremely busy.[28]

Pet therapy

Companion animals have been described as potentially fulfilling a number of functions for older people with dementia. They can be objects of affection, empathy and communication, as well as a focal point for group communications and activities in residential care. Benefits may extend to staff, caregivers and volunteers as well. Socialisation may be improved. Pets do not suit everybody so it is important to identify those who have an aversion to a particular animal. As we all know, there are 'cat people' and 'dog people'. There are also potential dangers, with the possibility of falls due to tripping over an animal being a major concern, and the need to supervise well-meaning efforts to care for an animal that may inadvertently harm it. There is very little evidence of pet therapy being effective.[29]

Light therapy

It has been postulated that the commonly observed worsening of agitated behaviour in the late afternoon and early evening ('sundowning') may be partially due to changes in circadian sleep–wake cycles. The application of bright fluorescent lights for several hours during the day in an effort to influence these circadian rhythms was reported to have a modest effect on these behaviours in nursing home settings. However, a recent Cochrane Collaboration review concluded that there is insufficient evidence to assess the value of light therapy in dementia care.[30]

Multisensory stimulation – Snoezelen rooms

Multisensory stimulation has become very popular in the UK as a treatment for calming agitation, stimulating those who are withdrawn and encouraging communication with caregivers. It was initially used for people with learning disabilities but over the last 15 years has also been used in dementia care. The Snoezelen room is a plain room without adornment, with white or cream walls, ceiling and carpet. With the room light dimmed, multisensory equipment projects glowing colours through fibre optics and tubes of water that results in moving bubbles. Pleasing nature scenes or abstract patterns are projected on the walls. Mirror balls resurrected from the disco era are slowly rotated to produce small coloured dots. Quiet, calming music is played in the background and aromatherapy might be used as well to stimulate the sense of smell. As a caregiver accompanies the person with dementia, touch and communication are encouraged as they explore the various effects. Usually sessions are of about 30 minutes duration and held twice weekly on a one-to-one basis.

Research into this therapy is very limited and it is unclear whether there are any benefits over and above what might accrue from an activity programme. There are reports that some people have improvements in social behaviour and communication up to a month after therapy has ended. Some individuals respond very well; however, others are unable to tolerate the environment and may become very distressed. There is really insufficient evidence for the widespread use of this approach.[31]

Physical restraints

The use of physical restraints in dementia care is not recommended. They used to be widespread in aged care facilities but this fortunately seems to have diminished in recent years. Although the reasons given for using restraints might sound reasonable, for example, to prevent falls in a person unable to ambulate safely, there is little evidence that they are effective in doing this. Others are used to prevent wandering. The most commonly used restraints are the Posey, which is worn as a type of vest and tied to a chair, the lap belt that is also tied to a chair, a tray table placed in front of a chair, and raised cotsides.

There are numerous problems with restraints. First, most restrained people become more agitated because they are uncomfortable. Behavioural disturbances usually worsen. Second, some restraints are dangerous, particularly lap restraints that have been known to strangle older people who slip down from the chair. Others may cause circulatory problems.

Third, many are applied as a consequence of inadequate staffing levels rather than as an appropriate response to a clinical problem. This often has the corollary of meaning that staff inadequately monitor the restraints. Fourth, too often restraints are applied without obtaining appropriate consent.

There are some situations where restraints might be appropriate, for example, an acutely sick person with dementia who keeps pulling out catheters may need to be temporarily restrained, although safe alternative strategies are available. In residential care some agitated people with dementia become calmer at mealtimes with a tray table in front of them. These should be the exceptions rather than the rule.

Summary

Psychosocial and other treatments for dementia are largely about assisting the person with dementia and their caregivers live with the disease with the best possible quality of life. This is very similar to the holistic approaches used in other chronic illnesses. By concentrating on abilities rather than disabilities and by providing an emotionally supportive environment, psychosocial treatments allow the person with dementia to function at an optimal level.

Family and Other Caregivers

Dementia has an enormous impact upon family and friends. Living with a person with dementia is often very stressful, particularly as the dementia progresses into the moderate and severe stages and as personality and behavioural changes become more apparent. Observing the gradual decline of a loved one from a competent individual to an incompetent dependent can be a harrowing experience. The demands upon the time and emotions of those providing care – the caregivers – can be huge.[1] A famous book written about caregiving in the mid-1980s by Nancy Mace and Peter Rabins was entitled *The 36-hour Day*.[2] The title said it all for so many caregivers and it instantly became a bestseller worldwide. However caregiving is not all negative, and in this chapter I consider some of the positive aspects too.

The impact of early dementia

Pre-diagnosis

In previous chapters I have described how the early symptoms of dementia may be non-specific and are often attributed to other causes. Depending on the type of symptoms that predominate, the early impact of dementia upon family and friends is quite variable. There is little doubt, however, that spouses and others living with the person with dementia experience the greatest impact.

> *Jim and his 74-year-old wife Penny lived a quiet, happy life. Jim first noticed that Penny was becoming forgetful when she kept losing her house keys. Initially it was a source of humour between them but when it happened repeatedly over a six-month period, Jim became aware that Penny was also forgetting telephone conversations and visits to friends,*

and she was leaving the stove on. Penny was also retreating from her previous standards of household cleanliness and seemed more reliant on Jim to help around the house. This didn't bother Jim too much and he just put the memory lapses down to age. But what did bother him was Penny's increasing reluctance to allow him to spend his usual hour or two with his mates at the club a few days a week. She became very anxious and fearful that something would happen whilst he was away. Jim couldn't understand the change, as this had been a life-long habit that Penny had always been content about. It was Penny's anxiety and Jim's mounting frustration with the restrictions upon his lifestyle that resulted in him taking Penny, upon the advice of his son, to their local doctor to discuss the problem. Their doctor quickly cottoned on to Penny's forgetfulness and that this was likely to be part of an early dementia, but it was the first time that Jim had considered that the forgetfulness and anxiety were linked.

This case illustrates that it is often not memory changes that cause the greatest concern early on, particularly when the caregiver does not recognise the symptoms as being abnormal. The point when lifestyle changes are forced upon the caregiver is often the point when help is requested. These days, however, more and more people are becoming aware that memory changes may be due to dementia, and it is increasingly common for the spouse to become concerned at the earliest signs of memory decline and therefore arrange an assessment. For children with parents who live alone, the impact of mild dementia in their parent can present them with a number of conflicts, as illustrated in the following case.

Rachel was an organised woman. Married to Tom, a professional with a busy career, and the mother of three teenage children, she needed to be organised to fit in her part-time job as a teacher. Her widowed mother, Rose, lived nearby and, being the eldest daughter, Rachel had always felt obligated to her. Over a period of 18 months, Rachel became aware that her mother's faculties were failing. Previously completely independent, Rose now needed to be reminded to pay her bills and was unable to do her shopping by herself. Rachel naturally stepped in to help and, before she knew it, was doing all of her mother's shopping, managing her finances and preparing many of her meals. It was not long before Rachel started to feel burdened by her various roles, particularly when her husband started to grumble that he wasn't seeing her. She also felt bitter towards her younger brother, who couldn't understand why she was concerned and was not making any effort to help. It was these pressures that led Rachel to seek help from the local aged care service. Through them a dementia assessment was arranged and community support services organised.

It was only at the family meeting during the assessment that Rachel's husband and brother finally started to recognise the extent of the problem and Rachel's need for support.

Facing the diagnosis

As I noted in Chapter 6, the dementia assessment process should provide family members with the opportunity to come to grips with the diagnosis and start planning for the future. Most family members will have already anticipated the worst, having realised that there was something seriously wrong long before the person with dementia was aware of any concerns. But some family members may also have greater difficulty in initially accepting the news. Possibly the prospect of living with a person with confirmed dementia is different to living with person who is 'a bit forgetful'. The future may suddenly appear bleaker as worst fears are confirmed: 'How will I cope with looking after him/her?' The spouse may worry about the chances that the children will be at risk of dementia; the children may worry about themselves and their own children: 'Am I going to get dementia?' 'When do we have to start looking for a nursing home?' All of these and other concerns may crowd in.

Family concerns about the genetic risk posed to children and grandchildren are common. It should be remembered, as was discussed in Chapter 3, that with late-onset Alzheimer's disease there is less than 10 per cent chance that a first-degree relative (child or sibling) will develop Alzheimer's disease before the age of 78, and for second-degree relatives such as grandchildren this probably drops to less than 5 per cent risk.[3] With younger-onset Alzheimer's disease and frontotemporal dementia the situation is quite different, as discussed below. Most other types of dementia have some degree of genetic influence, but there is less research data to provide families with accurate estimates of risk. In general, though, families can be largely reassured about their own risks of developing dementia.

Early decisions

Many family members and persons with dementia are well aware of the 'memory drugs' (cholinesterase inhibitors) and are keen to commence treatment. Imagine the disappointment that some families experience to be told that their relative does have dementia, but the drugs are not suited for their type of dementia, or that they have a health problem that makes the treatment too risky. Sometimes these drugs are used 'off-label' for

conditions where the FDA and other national drug regulatory authorities have not approved their use. But caution is needed as in some types of dementia, such as frontotemporal dementia, there is good evidence that the cholinesterase inhibitors are ineffective and should not be used.[4]

As far as possible, it is desirable that the person with dementia chooses the family members they wish to participate in their decision-making. Sometimes family conflicts or geographical separation (children interstate or overseas) prevent this from happening effectively, but there are often ways to get around difficulties. Email and videoconferencing over the internet are effective ways for rural, interstate and overseas children to communicate with other family members and doctors about their parents. In general, the types of early decisions that need to be made relate to financial management (enduring power of attorney, making a will), driving and possibly enduring guardianship, all described in detail in Chapter 12. All such decision-making is assisted by family education about dementia in general, with specific information about the type of dementia which has been diagnosed. Usually there is no need to discuss the potential need for nursing home placement at this early stage, but some families do seek particular information. I usually direct family members to the Alzheimer's Association, contactable either by phone or the internet, to get more information (see Appendices 1 and 2) and suggest they join the Association's caregiver support groups.

In mild dementia it is desirable that families try to live as normally as possible. In many areas there will be no need to make major lifestyle changes. However, if the person with dementia or the family have particular ambitions or plans to take a specific holiday trip or take up a new pastime, then it is 'now or never'. Meeting some ambitions may already be beyond the capacity of the person with dementia, such as undertaking a university course, but many other things are still quite achievable and most are desirable. Nostalgia trips to childhood and adolescent neighbourhoods are popular, particularly for migrants.

Issues in younger-onset dementia
The baby boomer generation is currently aged in their 50s and early 60s and due to this population bulge there has been an upsurge in the number of persons with younger-onset dementia, pragmatically defined as dementia commencing under the age of 65. When a younger person develops dementia, the family impact can be devastating from a number of perspectives. The diagnosis of any serious, incurable illness is harder to

deal with in a younger person than in old age largely because such illnesses are 'out of phase' with what most of us expect to happen at that life stage. This is much more the case with dementia, not only due to its very nature, but also because it is very much a disease of old age. The life plans of the person with dementia and their families are permanently disrupted.[5]

Younger people with dementia are likely to be in the workforce, and usually the dementia will mean early retirement. Unless they have been contributing to a good superannuation scheme or have disability insurance, this often means a significant reduction in family income with all its associated ramifications, including mortgage and debt repayments, and lifestyle changes. Where a spouse retires early to look after a partner with dementia, there may be a similar effect.

It is also more likely that the person with dementia will have children still at home. The effect of living with a parent with dementia may be overwhelming, and there are some very moving testimonials written by school-age children. There are some good fictionalised accounts too. In her famous 1929 novel *Ultima Thule* – the final volume in *The Fortunes of Richard Mahony* trilogy – Australian author Henry Handel Richardson drew on her experiences of living with her father with dementia when she was a child.[6] The effects of her father's cognitive and behavioural changes upon the family are described in graphic detail.[7]

To some extent, the degree to which children cope with the situation depends on how well the other parent is coping. But that is to oversimplify the situation. Even when the other parent is present and is coping well, children need special attention to help them understand what is happening. The type of support children need varies with their age, particularly in terms of how best to provide explanation. Fortunately Alzheimer's Associations have publications for children that can assist;[8, 9] the involvement of child and adolescent counselling services is usually helpful.

Another difficult issue with younger onset dementia is the increased likelihood that the dementia may be hereditary. As described in Chapters 3 and 5, some dementias in this age group may have a 50 per cent chance of being transmitted to offspring. This is particularly likely if there have been three or more first-degree family members with a dementia diagnosis. In these circumstances genetic counselling is advisable. Predictive genetic testing is advisable, but there is at least a 30 per cent chance that no genetic mutation will be found. In the absence of any treatments to prevent the expression of the dementia if a mutation were found, most people do not want to know and the take-up for predictive testing is low.[10]

If placement becomes a consideration later in the course of dementia, most families will find that there are few if any residential facilities that suit the younger person with dementia. Over half of the residents in aged care facilities are aged 85 years and over, so a person in their 40s or 50s usually feels out of place. This difficulty can mean much unneeded added stress to those affected by younger-onset dementia. I am leading a collaboration of researchers from Sydney, Australia (the Inspired Study) that is examining the needs of younger persons with dementia and their families with the view to determining the most appropriate models of service delivery.[11] Our early results suggest that no single model will fit the diverse range of conditions that cause younger onset dementia.

The impact of moderate dementia

As described in Chapter 4, in the moderate stage of dementia the person with dementia requires some level of assistance from other people to enable them to maintain their function in the community at a level as near as possible to the level they enjoyed before the onset of the dementia. It is often in this stage that caregivers begin to realise the full extent of the various demands upon their time.[12] While the deteriorating memory function is a problem, it is usually not the main feature of dementia that impacts upon the caregiver. It is more often the personality and behavioural changes that cause the most concern, with these changes having the greatest effect on those caregivers who live with the person with dementia, usually the spouse. During this stage of dementia, not only does it become very difficult for the person with dementia to live independently, but it also becomes very difficult for the co-resident caregiver to have a life of his or her own.

What types of demands are placed upon the caregiver? The following examples give some indication.

Max had suffered from vascular dementia for three years. As his dementia worsened, he began to wake up regularly through the night. For a while his wife Doreen was able to settle him, and he would sleep fitfully for a few more hours. Eventually, he would regularly awaken at around 3am, convinced that it was morning and time to go to work. No amount of persuasion from Doreen could convince him otherwise as he dressed and demanded his breakfast. To avoid conflict she would have to get up and pretend for an hour or so to help him go to work before she was able to distract him by putting on the television.

Every few minutes Vicki would ask her husband, Pete, when they were going out to their daughter's home. He would reply as calmly as he could that they were leaving in two hours as their daughter was still at work. After an hour of this had passed, he started to get quite frustrated and decided to leave early. Once they were there, every few minutes Vicki would ask when they would be going home. This pattern recurred daily, much to Pete's consternation.

Tony had always been a walker, a habit that didn't change as his dementia progressed. He would be out every morning for a couple of hours, walking around his neighbourhood. His wife, Karen, was increasingly concerned about Tony's safety, particularly as he seemed so confused at home at the best of times, and on the occasions he was out with her at the shops he seemed oblivious to his surroundings. One morning he failed to return at his usual time and Karen was really worried. She searched the immediate neighbourhood without success. Five hours later the local police brought him home – he had been found wandering along the side of a motorway, obviously lost. To prevent this happening again, Karen decided it would be easier for her to walk with Tony every morning herself than trying to stop his life-long habit.

Disrupted sleep patterns, repetitive questioning and wandering are three examples of behaviours that place demands upon the caregiver's time and cause enormous strain or burden.[13, 14] Some of these behaviours require extra supervision from the caregiver, especially the sleep changes and wandering, increasing the demands on their time and requiring them to be vigilant even when they need time for themselves to relax. Some other types of behavioural and personality change, including aggressive outbursts and paranoid accusations, have a greater impact upon the actual relationship between the person with dementia and caregiver and can threaten the wellbeing of the caregiver. (Examples of such situations appear in Chapter 4.) When the fundamental basis of a relationship is being undermined by such behaviours, even the most empathic, understanding and tolerant caregiver may come to a breaking point. Fortunately, these behaviours are far from universal, and in many cases may improve with medical and psychosocial strategies described in previous chapters. Probably the most important way of helping caregivers deal with these problems is through family education and support, as described later in this chapter.

Abuse of people with dementia by caregivers

Occurring in a minority of cases, abuse of the person with dementia by the caregiver is one of the negative consequences of caregiving that tends to emerge in the moderate stage of dementia.[15] While elder abuse occurs in the general population, persons with dementia are at increased risk. Most perpetrators of abuse live with the victim and deliver a significant amount of care. Caregivers who admit to abuse are more likely than non-abusers to have a history of mental illness and alcohol abuse. They are also more likely to report that they have been physical abused by the person with dementia, often for many years before the dementia developed. It is generally accepted that there are basically two groups of abusive caregivers.

The first group consists of bona fide caregivers who are under enormous stress and get caught up in a cycle of despair. These caregivers really need support and respite from their circumstances as discussed later in this chapter and in Chapter 10. Usually, home care can continue once these issues have been addressed.[16]

The second group has been labelled as 'pathological caregivers'; they perpetrate serious abuse as part of a lifestyle of violence, sociopathic behaviour and abuse of drugs and alcohol. In these cases other abusive behaviours, including sexual abuse and financial abuse, are more likely to be present. The only reasonable solution is protection of the person with dementia, which generally means permanent separation from the caregiver. The dilemma here is that this often means placement into residential care, and the person with dementia will frequently state a preference to remain at home, despite the abuse, to avoid placement.[17] In Australia, the regional Aged Care Assessment Team (ACAT) is the main agency responsible for the investigation and management of elder abuse. Often the ACAT has to apply for a public guardian to be appointed to ensure that appropriate decisions are made on behalf of the person with dementia (see Chapter 12).

The impact of severe dementia

In severe dementia, as described in Chapter 4, there is no semblance of independent function so maintenance at home usually requires 24-hour care from family, friends and community support services. This involves assistance with all basic activities of daily living (ADLs) – feeding, toileting, dressing, bathing and grooming. In addition, the behavioural changes previously described tend to persist and often worsen before there is a

diminution as the dementia becomes more advanced. The following case typifies the impact upon the caregiver.

> Adele was looking after her husband Philip, who had severe Alzheimer's disease. Her daily routine began around 6am when Philip awoke and noisily started to try to dress himself. Without her help he would usually put on his clothes inside out, or try to put his arms through the trouser legs, getting himself into a frustrated mess. Breakfast followed and of course she would have to monitor his feeding, make sure he got the cereal into his mouth, that his toast was cut and that his tea was not too hot. Then she would try to entice him to have a wash and allow her to shave him so that he could be ready to be picked up by the day centre bus at around 9.30am. When he was at the day centre — two days a week — Adele would take the opportunity to do her shopping and have some time with friends. This was really the only time she had to relax apart from periods at the weekend when her daughter would help out. For the rest of the time, she had to be with Philip constantly, as he could no longer be left alone for more than a few minutes. He had a tendency to wander and had got lost several times already. Fortunately Philip remained a placid man who could still show affection, even though his speech was now very limited. This helped Adele to keep going.

When physical ailments are also present, the burden upon the caregiver is amplified.

> Richard had severe vascular dementia. He had just suffered another stroke and was now unable to walk without assistance. His memory was very poor and he was often disoriented. He wet the bed every night and needed assistance from his wife, Cindy, to shower and dress. Richard was a heavy man and Cindy quite petite; despite her best efforts and the assistance of community nurses, it was clear to all of the health professionals involved that Cindy was unlikely to cope much longer. When advised to place her husband into a nursing home, Cindy vehemently refused. Intellectually, she understood that she was at the limits of her ability to look after Richard. Emotionally, she could not bear to part from her confidant. It was only when Richard had yet another stroke that the hospital geriatrician and social worker were able to convince her that placement was the best option.

It is usually during this stage of dementia that families have to grapple with the difficult task of placement; it might come earlier if the person with dementia lives alone. This is often an emotionally distressing period for caregivers, especially if the caregiver has been determined to look after the person with dementia at home until they die. The reality is that very few

caregivers are able to achieve this ambition; 24-hour care is enormously difficult to provide over a period of some years, even with the involvement of community services. Those fortunate enough to be able to self-fund 24-hour personal care assistants to take the load off their shoulders are more likely to achieve it but the costs are prohibitive. I cover issues related to community services and residential care in Chapters 10 and 11.

The other major issue confronting caregivers by this stage of dementia is the grieving process.[18, 19] Anticipatory grief, in which a person begins to grieve before the death of a loved one, is particularly common in severe dementia due to the premature loss of many of the personal attributes, otherwise known as the 'self', upon which the relationship was based, but it is also a significant factor contributing to caregiver stress earlier in the dementia. When your loved one no longer recognises you, is generally incoherent and lives in a nursing home it is little wonder that it seems as if they have died. For some caregivers, the grieving process may be virtually completed before the person with dementia's death. This often results in cessation of visits to the nursing home and irritation about being asked to remain involved. For other caregivers, anticipatory grief has the effect of drawing out the grieving process for a much longer period than with many other terminal illnesses, resulting in a chronic period of heightened emotions that may take years to resolve even after the death.

Jonathan Franzen, author of the novel *The Corrections*,[20] has written about the death of his father from Alzheimer's disease. He comments on how he had been mourning his father for years before he died. He also notes that even in the advanced stage of dementia when his father could no longer recognise him, he felt compelled to look for meaning in his father's existence and was surprised that he kept finding it.[21] This search for meaning is an experience common to many caregivers.

Caregiver burden and depression

The concept of caregiver burden includes the objective practical problems caregivers face in day-to-day care, as has been described in the preceding paragraphs, and the subjective strain or emotional reaction that caregivers experience that might include symptoms of stress, depression and anxiety.[22] Caregivers have high rates of depression with some studies finding over 40 per cent of caregivers meet diagnostic criteria for clinical depression. Interventions to prevent caregiver stress and depression are described later in the chapter and of course are paramount in any caregiver support

strategy. It is also important, however, to ensure that caregiver depression is adequately assessed and treated. Untreated depression results in much suffering, caregivers are unable to function optimally, and there is the added risk of suicide. Usually the caregiver's doctor is the best starting point for assessment, though some people prefer to access their local mental health service first. In general, standard treatments for depression (psychotherapies and/or antidepressant medication) are effective, with the type of treatment determined by the severity and clinical features of the depression.

Gender differences

In general, female caregivers seem to have higher levels of distress than male caregivers.[23] There are many theories about this. Certainly, women in our society are more likely to be thrust into the caregiving role than men, so they may feel obligated, and as though they have less choice in the matter than men do. Female caregivers are also more likely to be 'hands-on' caregivers – that is, they tend to do everything themselves rather than delegate to others. Male caregivers tend to have more of a 'managerial' style that allows them to distance themselves a bit more from the stressful situation to some degree by delegating tasks.

Another factor contributing to the differential experience of stress relates to the psychological development of, and social roles fulfilled by, men and women at different stages of the life cycle.[24] Historically, women have tended to have a nurturing and caring role in their early to mid-adult life for child rearing. When the children grew up, women tended to pursue their personal development through a delayed career or other interests. A return to a primary nurturing and caring role may not fit in with many women's later life plans. In contrast, men have tended to be in the workforce during their early to mid-adult life and have not had much of a nurturing role. As they age, men's psychological development turns to a more nurturing role, best exemplified by the grandfather who spends more time with his grandchildren than he ever did with his children. Thus, for some older men, the nurturing role of caregiving may be more in keeping with their personal development than it is for some older women.

Family education and support

Education about dementia is an essential component of helping families live with a person with dementia. At its simplest level, initial education may involve the provision of information about the type of dementia, its

course, what to expect, plans to make and the treatments available. This might be delivered at the time of diagnosis by the assessment team, or by books, brochures and the internet. Information about specific problems such as behavioural changes may be needed as the circumstances arise. But knowledge alone is usually insufficient as demonstrated in a few studies.

In one of the major studies in this field in the late 1980s, Professor Henry Brodaty, with Meredith Gresham, developed a caregivers training programme at Prince Henry Hospital in Sydney. The structured, intensive ten-day residential programme involved a mix of education, skills training and stress management as a package delivered early in the course of dementia. After the period of initial training, ongoing emotional support was provided in groups and by teleconferences. The design of the study compared three randomly allocated groups. The first group of caregivers received the training programme immediately; the second group was placed on a 'wait list' and received the programme six months later; the third group received ten days of respite care. During the period of the programme, each of the people with dementia received a ten-day structured memory training and activity programme. The study found that caregiver stress was significantly lower in those caregivers who received the training. Just as importantly, the benefits persisted. The earlier in the course of dementia that a caregiver received the training package, the greater the perceived benefit. One of the surprising findings was that benefits appeared to persist for up to eight years. Nursing home placement was delayed and, quite unexpectedly, survival of the person with dementia was longer. This survival was not simply related to delays in nursing home placement and could not be explained by any particular features of the person's dementia.[25]

There is now a growing body of research that has demonstrated the benefits of family education and support, though attempts to identify the critical components of the various training programmes that have been used by various groups around the world have not been very successful.[26] Further, training programmes do not suit everybody. There is some evidence that suggests that while early intervention is important, caregivers also need to be ready for the intervention. If the family member feels in control of the situation and does not feel under any stress, they may not feel that attending a programme is of much use at that time and would rather wait until they feel it is necessary. In other cases, readiness to undertake training may be related more to the caregiver's psychological preparedness to deal with the problem than to any sense of being in control. Caregivers who

are feeling stressed and are looking for some answers probably obtain the greatest benefit from this type of programme. The Alzheimer's Association in Australia has developed a 'Living with memory loss' programme that includes both caregivers and the person with early dementia separately in a course of group sessions along these lines.

Most research in the field of caregiving has focused on the primary caregiver and paid little attention to other family members. This has been particularly the case when other family members live interstate or overseas. There is mounting evidence, however, that the involvement of as many family members as possible within the education and support process is beneficial. Frequently the designated primary caregiver, for example the spouse, can only effectively fulfil that role with the active support of other family members such as children or siblings. By including these other family members in the educational and support programme, it is more likely that the primary caregiver will receive support. Individuals within the one family, however, may have different degrees of preparedness and willingness to participate in caregiver training programmes and may not wish to participate all at the same time. Often, however, important issues arise that can only be effectively dealt with in the family group, especially when individual family members have differing opinions about what should happen. Conflict most commonly emerges during the period when institutional care is being considered. Other issues that may be the basis for conflict include financial management and the use of medications.

Alzheimer's Associations

Alzheimer's Associations are the peak consumer and caregiver non-government organisations in most countries. Worldwide there are Alzheimer's Associations in over one hundred countries, most of which belong to Alzheimer's Disease International that coordinates efforts and organises an annual international conference. Alzheimer's Associations provide information about dementia to caregivers, persons with dementia and the general public and often organise support services for caregivers. Some Alzheimer's Associations are very politically active in lobbying their governments for more funding for services and research.

In Australia, the critical role that Alzheimer's Australia has played in lobbying governments to improve services for dementia care cannot be overemphasised. Politicians listen more to consumers than health professionals about service requirements, and the cogent arguments and

submissions provided by Alzheimer's Australia has seen funding flow to a range of projects that include 24-hour telephone helplines for caregivers, caregiver education programmes including those for caregivers of various ethnic groups, programmes for people with early dementia, caregiver respite programmes and various caregiver support groups. Most services involved with dementia care in Australia have developed strong links with their local Alzheimer's Association. In many cases they supply the group leaders for their local caregiver support groups. Details of how to contact Alzheimer's Associations are listed in Appendices 1 and 2.

Positive aspects of caregiving

Caregiving should not be characterised only by its negative attributes. Many caregivers report heightened feelings of love and affection for the person with dementia, which have arisen from their caregiving experience. The relationship may become closer with the sharing of life experiences that might not have otherwise occurred. There is often a sense of reciprocation in which caregivers feel they are repaying an emotional debt to the person with dementia. This is particularly the case with adult children who feel their parent has made sacrifices for them.

> When Michael's wife Sarah was diagnosed with Alzheimer's disease just short of her 75th birthday, Michael was determined that she would be well looked after. Married for 55 years, they had experienced a number of ups and downs but they had always pulled through. Michael felt that Sarah deserved his care and attention; for one thing, he had never forgotten the support that she provided him when he returned injured after the Korean War. In more recent years, she had helped him pull through a cancer scare. Michael was diligent in finding out about all of the community services available to assist dementia caregivers but reasoned that he would only call on them when needed. Despite having to learn how to cook and forever having difficulty with his ironing, Michael seemed to thrive. He made use of the dementia day care centre each week and found the time that this availed him to be sufficient to get his chores done. He kept in touch with his mates and was still fortunate that he could get out to the club for a few hours each week with Sarah. She enjoyed this and Michael was constantly surprised how 'normally' she could behave.

Caregiving is full of challenges and for many caregivers it brings an opportunity to broaden their life experiences, albeit not necessarily in the way they had planned. Personal growth may be attained through the mastery of new skills and better self-awareness. For example, a

caregiver might have to learn about financial management or household management, both of which can bring the caregiver a sense of achievement. In relationships where the caregiver has been subservient to a domineering partner, increased personal autonomy may occur as the caregiver gradually gains confidence to more fully express themselves.

Summary

Dementia has a major impact upon the person with dementia's family and friends. Family caregivers take up the brunt of the burden of care in mild and moderate dementia; by the time the dementia is severe, however, most have reached the end of their tether and have had to place the person with dementia into residential care. Despite this, many caregivers report positive experiences from caregiving. Alzheimer's Associations worldwide have developed as the primary consumer organisations for support of caregivers and persons with dementia.

CHAPTER 10

Community Care Services

Most people would probably state a preference to live at home until they die. Most families would probably prefer to look after their disabled relatives for as long as possible at home. However, because dementia is such a slowly progressive condition, by comparison with other illnesses such as cancer, the time frame over which care needs to be provided is very long. Without a strong community care system, most families and other caregivers are hamstrung in their efforts to look after the person with dementia at home.

History of community care

The provision of community-based services to support people living with disabilities in their own home is standard practice these days and so it is easy to forget that it is a relatively recent style of service delivery. It is only since World War II that community-based services started to appear; before that institutional care was the only type of service available for the care of people with chronic mental and physical disabilities when the burden of care was beyond the limits of their families and friends, or when the person had no one to look after them. Changes started to appear in the 1950s in the UK and the 1960s in the US and in both countries were at least partially fuelled by concerns about the increasing costs of institutional care of older people and the belief that community care was not only cheaper but preferable for most people as it improved their quality of life.[1, 2] For many conditions, such as severe mental illness and Parkinson's disease, the move to community care was also facilitated by better medical treatments that enabled disabled people to live relatively independently in the community with support services instead of in long-term hospitals and nursing homes. In most countries the development of

community services to support older disabled people with dementia has been a long, slow evolution that remains a 'work in progress'. I will briefly examine service developments in the UK, the US and Australia.

UK

In the UK, while community care had been gradually developing since the 1950s, it was not until the 1986 Audit Commission report, 'Making Reality of Community Care', outlined the advantages of home-based care that it became the government's policy of care.[3] The government then commissioned the 1988 Griffiths Report that set out to define the boundaries between health and social services. The report recommended that social services in local authorities should have the key role in long-term and continuing community care while the National Health Service (NHS) should be responsible for health care. A subsequent government white paper in 1989, which was enacted in 1990 and became operational in 1993, included development of needs assessment and case management, promotion of domiciliary, day and respite care, and provision of practical support for caregivers.[4, 5] In effect this made social service departments gatekeepers that control access to government-funded community services based upon need. Need could be in any of six broad domains – personal/social care, health care, accommodation, finance, education/employment/leisure, or transport/access. A single assessment process is used to assess these needs, and for older people one of the areas that has to be covered is cognition and dementia. This process should follow a personalised approach in which the person being assessed and their caregiver are at the centre of the decision-making process about what services are needed and how they might be delivered.

There are mixed views on the effects of these changes in the UK over the last 20 years with a general consensus that there is chronic underfunding and a lack of coalface interface between health and social services.[6, 7] The importance of the latter is that because an older person with cognitive problems does not need to have a formal diagnosis of dementia, unless there is a good interface between social and health services, an adequate dementia assessment by a health professional might not occur in a timely fashion. Even the release of the UK's dementia strategy in 2009 did not appease some critics.[8] Another problem has been the failure to assess for dementia at all. A July 2012 All Party Parliamentary Group on Dementia report – *Unlocking Diagnosis: The Key to Improving the Lives of People with Dementia* – recommended that health and social care professionals should

routinely ask questions to identify symptoms of dementia in all 'at risk' people.[9]

US

Community service development in the US has followed a different approach in which state-funded services are means-tested, leaving a greater reliance on self-funding and long-term care insurance. The 1965 establishment of Medicare that focuses on acute care, and Medicaid that focuses on long-term care, were ground breaking at the time. Medicaid is a means-tested programme with co-payments that funds long-term care in both the community and institutions but there are significant gaps in coverage. A third programme established in 1965 under the Older Americans Act for low-income elders promotes social services including home care and meals programmes through state agencies and non-government organisations.[10] After this initial burst of development little government-funded innovation of community services occurred until the 1990s. In the 1980s private companies introduced Elder Care Assistance Programs, paralleling those developed to support workers with young children. These included resource and referral services to locate care services for older people in their community, and flexible spending accounts for putting aside funds on a pre-tax basis to cover elder care expenses.

The next major public community service innovation started in 1990 when Medicaid and Medicare co-funded Programmes of All-inclusive Care of the Elderly (PACE) in which an interdisciplinary team assesses the needs of Medicaid-eligible older people, develops care plans, and delivers all services (including acute care services and nursing facility services when necessary), which are integrated for a seamless provision of total care.[11, 12] Again these services are means-tested. Public funded support for caregivers did not really appear until 1993 when the Family and Medical Leave Act gave caregivers 12 weeks of job protected unpaid leave if they worked for an eligible company, which is approximately 55 per cent of the workforce. The National Family Caregiver Support Program, which was introduced in 2000, offers services such as respite care, counselling and caregiver training, but there are concerns that it has only limited funding.[13]

Australia

In the early 1980s, serious questions began to be asked about the direction of Australian Commonwealth Government funding for aged care. With the ageing population, government funding for nursing homes was spiralling

out of control while very little was being invested into community services to support older people in their own homes.

The 1986 landmark Nursing Home and Hostel Review set the ball into motion for change with an Aged Care Reform Strategy.[14] The four basic philosophical tenets underpinning the review were: to provide support to older and disabled people in their own homes; to provide residential services to older and disabled people only where their needs are not appropriately met by other support systems; for services to have a rehabilitation focus to restore function in a manner that develops and enhances personal freedom and independent functioning; and to recognise that for many older and disabled people, less supported residential services or community-based support services will be a possible and desirable outcome.

Apart from setting up the forerunners of the current Aged Care Assessment Teams, which in Australia are the gatekeepers that determine the eligibility of people for government-subsidised institutional care and community services based upon their level of disability, the Aged Care Reform Strategy also set limits upon the number of nursing home beds that were to be funded, redirecting the funding to community-based services. Dementia was recognised as a major cause of disability that required institutional care, and funding for dementia-specific community services started to flow in the late 1980s. The Australian National Action Plan for Dementia Care was launched in 1992 and covered seven elements – assessment, services for people with dementia, services for carers, quality of care, community awareness, research, and policy and planning.[15] Over the last 20 years, the Australian community-care sector has grown enormously in each of these areas, with numerous demonstration projects being piloted, some of which have evolved into standard service delivery. Many are based on models from other countries adapted to Australian conditions.

Funding of community long-term care

Because of the limits to publicly funded services in the US, Canada and to a certain extent in the UK and Australia, there is an increasing reliance on other ways of funding community services. Long-term care insurance generally covers for community and residential care not provided by Medicare, Medicaid, the NHS or health insurance. Those being insured will have their health rated which will determine if they are regarded as a

reasonable insurance risk and how much they will pay. Other factors that influence the premium include age, the benefits to be paid, and the period the benefit will pay for. Clearly long-term care insurance has to be taken out before a person has dementia.

Self-funded long-term care can occur by choice or by default. Some choose to structure their investments in such a way that if they require to fund community and residential services for themselves or a partner, they can do so relatively easily. Of course it helps to be reasonably wealthy. For many this can become the default option that may involve whittling away resources until they qualify for means-tested services.

Types and organisation of community services

In the rest of this chapter I describe the various types of community services that are frequently utilised in supporting people with dementia. In Table 10.1 I have listed the various services that might be useful for supporting the person with dementia and their caregiver. Service organisation, accessibility, costs and eligibility vary from country to country, and even jurisdictions within each country, but the basic types of services that are available are much the same. Information about accessing community services in various countries can be found on websites listed in Appendix 2.

Probably the commonest way in which community services are arranged occurs when a person with dementia (or more likely their caregiver) decides to get one specific type of service, such as assistance with housework or home-delivered meals. Of course, having a housekeeper to look after such chores is a matter of convenience rather than necessity for many people. But for older people who are having difficulty in the more physical aspects of independent living, this type of community service is often the first one used.

Using the UK as an example of a predominantly government-funded system, the first step in the process is to obtain a community-care assessment from the local authority social services department. The assessment is usually undertaken in the person's home by one or more health professionals such as a social worker, occupational therapist or nurse. This needs assessment must take into account the wishes of the person being assessed, any difficulties the person has due to physical or mental impairments (e.g. problems climbing stairs, cooking, bathing), health care needs, housing needs, informal caregiving supports available from family and friends, and the needs of those who are caregivers to the

person. With the consent of the person being assessed, GPs are expected to provide relevant health information for the assessment.[16]

Table 10.1 Types of community services

Service	What they do
Home help	Housework, meal preparation (home-delivered or prepared on site), laundry, gardening, shopping, home maintenance
Personal care	Toileting, bathing, dressing and feeding
Home nursing	Dressings, medication supervision, health monitoring
Other	Community transport, home modifications, in-home respite
Dementia day care centres	These provide day care for people with dementia and provide respite for their caregivers
Community geriatric services	These are therapy centres that offer a range of health services that may include geriatricians, specialist geriatric nurses, social workers, speech therapists, physiotherapists, podiatrists, occupational therapists and other therapies for older people. Assessments are usually multidisciplinary and may occur in the person's home or at the community centre
Hospital-in-the-Home	Multidisciplinary services that provide home-based acute medical care as an alternative to hospital admission
Old age (geriatric) psychiatry services	Services that treat older people with mental health problems. In dementia care, their main involvement occurs in diagnostic assessment and if there are significant behavioural and psychological symptoms complicating the dementia

If the community-care assessment demonstrates that there is sufficient unmet need to warrant community services, the local authority should then provide a written plan that details the services to be provided and the goals of the service provision. The plan should also include information about who provides the services, when they are to be provided and a contact point if there are problems including if there is a need for a review. The plan should also provide information about service charges.

There are three broad types of services that could be offered – domiciliary, day and respite care. Domiciliary care includes home help

(including housework, laundry and shopping), home maintenance or modification, personal care (such as toileting, bathing, dressing and feeding), home nursing, meal preparation and home-delivered meals, and allied health (physiotherapy, podiatry, occupational therapy, speech therapy). Day-care services are those that take place outside of the person's home and include day centres, lunch clubs and day hospitals. Respite care includes day care and residential respite.

There are complicated rules about payments for services in the UK and they vary according to whether the person lives in Scotland, England or Wales and they may also vary between local authorities. In general, services are means-tested in England and Wales, while in Scotland, for those over 65, personal care services should be free. The local Citizens Advice Bureau should be able to advise individuals about these payments and the options available. More information about these payments is on their website.[17] The Citizens Advice Bureau can also provide advice to individuals whose community-care assessment determined that they do not have sufficient unmet need to qualify for community services.

It is particularly important for people from ethnic minority groups to have personalised care.

Antonia was an 83-year-old, single, non-English speaking woman of Greek descent who had lived alone since her sister died five years earlier. Gradually over a period of some years her niece noted that she had become increasingly forgetful and lonely. She would regularly lose her keys and her purse. Her home was neglected, as was her personal hygiene. She wore the same filthy dress every day. Her diet was poor and she had lost around 10kg over the previous few years. Following a community-care assessment, a care package was organised that took into account her Greek heritage. The package involved regular visits from a Greek-speaking woman who did some of the housework and encouraged Antonia to bathe and change her clothes a few times per week. She could also assist in preparing the occasional Greek meal that supplemented regular Meals on Wheels. Antonia was also taken out to a Greek social club each week and she really enjoyed the company. Over some months she became much happier and put on some weight.

When a person has multiple and more complex service needs, for example home care, assistance with personal care and medication management, a more common way in which community services are arranged is as a package of care, usually personalised to the individual needs of the person

with dementia. In general, individuals that require this level of community services would also qualify for long-term residential care.

In the US, Programs of All-inclusive Care for the Elderly (PACE) are designed for persons aged 55 years and over who have been certified as eligible for nursing home care by the appropriate state agency and are assessed as being able to live safely in the community with the help of PACE services. PACE programmes are not universal in the US, thus individuals need to live in an area serviced by a PACE.[18]

In contrast to the UK model of care, PACE programmes include primary and specialist medical care, hospital care, dentistry, pathology and radiology services, medical transportation, prescription drugs and emergency care in addition to the range of community services for the person with dementia and the caregiver as previously described. It is funded via Medicare and Medicaid to cover all medically necessary care and services. Individuals who qualify for Medicare have all their Medicare-covered services paid by Medicare, while those that qualify for Medicaid either pay nothing or a small monthly payment for the community service (long-term care) portion of the PACE. If the person does not qualify for Medicaid, a monthly premium is charged to cover for long-term care and Medicare Part D drugs.[19]

Caregiver respite services

Respite care is particularly important for both people with dementia and their caregivers. A number of types of respite care are available, ranging in duration from a few hours to a few months. Probably the most frequently utilised form of respite care is dementia day care. Usually this involves the person with dementia being picked up by bus between 9 and 10am to spend about four or five hours in a day centre before being returned home between 3 and 4pm. Day care benefits the person with dementia through the social and diversional activities provided. It benefits the caregiver by allowing a much-needed break. There may be a period of adjustment for the person with dementia to the day centre. They may need a lot of persuasion to go there initially, but this reluctance usually settles quickly. Sometimes the caregiver may need to accompany them for the first few times.

Some people with dementia absolutely refuse to leave their homes and a co-resident caregiver may well feel trapped. In these circumstances in-home respite, where a community worker stays at home with the person with dementia while the caregiver goes out, might work. This type of respite is

also useful for a non-English speaking person when the community worker speaks their language. Sometimes overnight respite can be arranged.

Residential respite care is usually provided in a residential aged care facility. In most cases this is alongside permanent residents, though there are some facilities that specialise in respite care. There is some debate in the literature about whether residential respite care may cause harm to the person with dementia by increasing their confusion and agitation, along with the likelihood that psychotropic medication will be required to settle them.[20] Certainly there are individual cases where the period of residential respite becomes quite traumatic both for the person with dementia and the caregiver. Occasions where the caregiver is summoned in the middle of the night to take home an extremely agitated person can be very disturbing for all concerned. In most cases, however, there are few dramas apart from the expected settling-in period of the first few days.

For some caregivers, residential respite care is a prelude to permanent placement. During the course of the respite admission a caregiver may indicate that they are unable to take the person with dementia home again. In my experience this is most likely to happen with a very stressed caregiver who has been putting off taking a period of respite for a long time and, with the taste of life as a non-caregiver, realises that they just can't put themselves through it all again. In these circumstances every effort is usually made to accommodate the situation by finding a permanent long-term placement, often in the same facility.

Old age (geriatric) psychiatry services

These are services that treat older people with mental health problems in the community. In dementia care, their main involvement occurs if there are significant behavioural and psychological symptoms complicating the dementia. This is very important because of the high likelihood that if the symptoms continue unchecked, the person with dementia may be prematurely placed in residential care. Apart from providing specialist treatment, aged care psychiatry services usually provide short to medium-term support for caregivers including some education about dealing with the problem. There is good evidence that when intensive case management is provided to these persons with dementia and their caregivers, caregiver stress is reduced along with risk for the person with dementia and there are improvements in function and socialisation. Sometimes brief hospital admission to an acute aged care psychiatry unit is necessary if the symptoms are severe.

Unfortunately, these services are unevenly provided around many countries. Some juridictions, such as the state of Victoria in Australia, have very comprehensive well-funded and resourced services. Others are poorly funded and resourced.

Hospital in the Home programmes

Numerous programmes that have been piloted around the world aim to reduce the need for hospital care for physically unwell older people by providing a geriatric outreach service into the older person's home. The outreach service usually includes a geriatrician, nurses, physiotherapists and social workers who work in collaboration with the local doctor. The types of problems these services are particularly suited to treat include respiratory, urinary and skin infections, mild cardiac problems, and soft tissue injuries after a fall. This might be initiated in the person's home following a referral from the local doctor; after an assessment in the local emergency department; or following a brief admission to hospital to facilitate early discharge. For people with dementia, hospital admission can be extremely traumatic with increased confusion and behavioural problems due to the illness and new environment. Home-based care can often reduce these complications and improve the outcome.

Summary

Community services are particularly important in supporting people with dementia and their caregivers at home. There is a broad range of services available that focus on providing accurate assessments, minimising the effects of disability, providing support to caregivers and determining eligibility to residential care. These processes of assessment are often confusing for health professionals and caregivers alike. The current trends in community services are to increase flexibility in care provision through innovative strategies.

Residential Long-term Care

Most people with dementia will be placed into residential care in the moderate to severe stage of their illness, despite the best efforts of caregivers and community services to support them at home. Caregiver stress is one of the major factors leading to the breakdown of community care, and this in turn is often related to the behavioural aspects of the dementia. Other factors include the demands of physical care, the health of the caregiver and the availability of community support. If the person with dementia lives alone, placement is likely to come sooner, as it is very difficult to provide overnight supervision in a community setting. In this chapter I cover:

- the preparation required for entering residential care

- the basic requirements of good residential care

- the different types of residential care for dementia.

Why does placement into residential care occur?

Often, placement occurs because insufficient professional and non-professional community support is available to alleviate the pressure on caregivers or to look after a single person with dementia in their own home. The reasons behind insufficient community support are principally economic. Although residential care is very expensive, the cost of providing safe, quality, home-based care to people with severe dementia is even more expensive. Most people with severe dementia require 24-hour supervision and it is often the overnight care that is the stumbling block. The cost of community services that could provide this level of supervision is huge. Some wealthy people are able to afford it but the average person cannot.

Residential care in this situation is really an economic solution to a difficult problem. This doesn't mean that we shouldn't be trying to further increase the community services that are available. At this stage, the actual point at which community service provision becomes economically unviable for quality care has yet to be determined. However, it should also be recognised that for some caregivers, no amount of extra support will allow them to cope with the person with dementia at home. In addition, there are some individuals that prefer to live in group accommodation, often because of the relative ease in obtaining social contact with other older people.

Preparation required for entering residential care

Placement into a residential long-term care facility is often a very stressful process for caregivers and the person with dementia. Very few people with dementia will go by choice. In my experience, the majority of older people who are keen to go into residential care are clinically depressed and feel that they are an unwanted burden upon their family. Others seem agreeable to the placement and don't make a fuss, but usually they are quietly unhappy about it. Some will be vocally adamant that they will not go into 'a home' and at times a guardianship order will be required to provide legal authority for the placement against the wishes of the person with dementia (see Chapter 12).

Some steps can be taken in an attempt to minimise the stresses for caregivers and sometimes for the person with dementia. Caregivers are advised to plan ahead from a reasonably early point in the process of the dementia by finding out about the various facilities in their area. Facilities are usually prepared to show people around by appointment. Usually it is just the caregivers who have a look, but occasionally an insightful person with dementia may wish to participate in the decision-making. Some facilities allow names to be placed on a waiting list even when there is no immediate plan for placement. I don't think there is much point in putting a person's name on a waiting list unless there seems to be a likelihood of placement within a year.

In Australia, and increasingly in other countries, there are basic criteria of day-to-day function that determine whether a person is disabled enough for residential long-term care and the type of care required.[1] All persons with moderate dementia would be disabled enough to be suitable for residential care, but this doesn't mean that they need to be placed because caregivers and community services are able to support many at home.

How do you choose the 'best' facility? This is very difficult and often local availability is the main factor. If the person with dementia is from a non-English speaking background, and particularly if they speak little English or have very strong religious or cultural beliefs, a facility that specifically caters for these needs is advisable. As there are relatively few such facilities, this may well mean that families will have to travel a significant distance to visit the person with dementia.

Otherwise, choice should be guided by three factors – facility condition and design, staff attitudes and knowledge, and the particular needs of the person with dementia. These are all covered later in this chapter. Advice from the health professionals involved in the care of the person with dementia (doctor, community nurse, geriatrician, old age psychiatrist) should assist in the process. Sometimes a particular facility might appear excellent, but the health professionals may advise that it does not meet the person with dementia's needs. If it is very important to the person with dementia or the caregiver to maintain their long-term doctor, check which facilities they visit. Quite often a new doctor will be needed when entering residential care. In many larger facilities in North America and Europe the medical care is provided by a doctor attached to the facility rather than by a visiting doctor, so it may not be possible to retain their long-term doctor.

Preparation also includes psychological adjustment to the placement process. For many caregivers, placement is seen as an admission of failure; they feel that they have let the person with dementia down, that they are selfish, that they are abandoning their loved one. These emotions are understandable but in most circumstances are not accurate reflections of what has been happening. Caregivers may need to work through these emotions with a counsellor to avoid inappropriate self-blame from developing. Other caregivers are able to see that they have done as much as they can to look after the person with dementia at home and are able to focus on the next step. Research shows that most caregivers adjust to the placement and after about six months are much less stressed than they were beforehand.

The person with dementia can often be gradually prepared for the placement by the caregiver and health professionals talking about the topic from time to time to gauge their receptivity. This may have to be subtle because some people are very sensitive about the issue and may flare up at the mere mention of residential placement. A method that works for some people is to use residential respite as a gradual introduction to

permanent placement. For others, an initial intention for temporary respite care may turn into permanent residential care without going home. In this regard, it is often noted that a person with dementia's outright opposition to placement disappears after being in residential care for a week or two, as illustrated in the following case.

> Christine lived alone and was supported by her only daughter Kay and a range of formal community support services. It was clear to all involved that despite their best efforts, Christine was becoming very unsafe at home. She would be up in the middle of the night and in her anxious confusion she would ring Kay repeatedly. During the day, she wandered from her home, and had to be brought home by the police on several occasions. Although Kay had considered taking her mother to live with her at her home, there really wasn't enough room and besides, Christine objected. She was equally vehement in her refusal to consider placement. After months of persuasion, and a fortuitous accident in which Christine flooded her kitchen, necessitating major repairs, Christine reluctantly agreed to a temporary placement until her kitchen was fixed. She was initially unsettled in the new environment but after a week she seemed quite content. Indeed, she commented to Kay 'how nice they all were'. After some weeks, during which time Christine made no mention of going back home, the respite placement was converted to a permanent placement.

Of course, there are many variants of this scenario. Another common outcome is for the person with dementia to remain unhappy about staying but no longer raising objections to it. In other cases, an unexpected medical complication develops, for example a stroke, and the combination of medical problems and dementia means community care is no longer feasible, even though there had previously been little time to plan for placement. Many people with dementia are placed into residential care from acute hospitals. One of the reasons for this is that it is generally easier to place a person when they are recovering from illness in an unfamiliar environment. Hospital doctors and nurses may more easily persuade the person with dementia at a time they are feeling less well in themselves and not up to self-care for a while.

Requirements of good residential care

There are two main requirements of good residential care. The first involves the delivery of quality professional health and personal care. The second involves ensuring that the residential care environment is as 'home like' as possible without compromising safety.

Professional health and personal care

The attitudes, knowledge and skills of the staff are probably the most important asset of any long-term care residential facility. The delivery of quality care requires well-trained staff that has a positive attitude towards older people with dementia and respects their rights. These two aspects of personal care – quality care and protection of resident rights – form the basis of legislated residential care standards in most countries including the UK, US, Canada, Australia and New Zealand.

Facilities vary in the level of professional supervision and personal care they provide. It is important for residents to retain as much autonomy as possible, so the degree of professional involvement varies according to functional need. Some facilities are intended to provide minimal levels of professional involvement for people who are functionally independent with limited supervision, while others are set up to provide high-level skilled nursing care for people fully dependent in their activities of daily living such as bathing, feeding and toileting. Of course, the less professional care required, the less expensive it is to run the facility, so financial considerations also influence the levels of care on offer; the funding source is keen to cap its costs. Occasionally some older people have the mistaken impression that they are going to be looked after as if they are in a hotel or private residence, with servants who are there to respond to their every wish. This often leads to conflicts with the staff, who resent being ordered around by a person capable of self-care.

There is a gradation of care from low to high-level depending on the individual needs of the resident as noted by the Aged Care Funding Instrument in Australia.[2] By the time a resident needs high-level care, health professional involvement, mainly skilled nursing, is required many times during the day. In all levels of care, specific training in dementia management is important though this can be difficult to achieve as many staff remain for only a few years. This is further complicated in most western countries by the high proportion of long-term care workers from culturally and linguistically diverse backgrounds who have difficulties in understanding English and may have trouble in appreciating cultural issues of the local residents.

There is a lot of research that has demonstrated very high stress levels in staff who work in long-term care facilities. Morale can become a problem in some facilities and low morale is often linked with suboptimal care.[3] In addition, with the current worldwide nursing shortages, many facilities are short staffed. Pay rates are also relatively low, so recruitment and retention of staff can be a problem.

Facility design and atmosphere

For many years, residential care design seemed to be dictated by staff and administrative considerations rather than the needs of residents, and so many facilities were sterile and institutional. Thankfully, designs over the last 20 years have improved considerably, with a better balance being achieved between the needs of staff, administrators, and residents, though costs often limit what can be done. This has been partially driven by more vigorous government standards for nursing home design, but also the belated recognition that long-term care facilities are the residents' homes.[4, 5] Despite these improvements, concern remains that fundamental design principles, which have been shown to be important to create the optimal environment for people with dementia, are not always being utilised in new facility developments. The reasons for this are unclear but can include not involving coalface nursing staff, who know what is required, in the planning process.

So, what design features are believed to assist in the care of people with dementia? One of the more important aspects of design is for it to be 'home-like'. The problem is that people come from diverse backgrounds and home conditions, thus there isn't a single design that fits all. This is amplified by our multicultural society, where the cultural traditions of different ethnic groups may be best met either by facilities specifically designed for one group, or by sections of a facility set aside for a particular group. Other reasons for needing culture-specific facilities include language, food, religion and other traditions.

Another design feature touted for dementia is 'age-appropriateness' whereby the facility is intended to remind the person with dementia of their younger adult days through the colour schemes, fittings and furnishings, on the presumption that this will put them more at ease. The dilemma here is that there may be a 40-year age spread among residents in the one facility, so its design might have to incorporate the interim from the 1920s to the 1960s, a period in which many home changes occurred. A person who might feel quite at ease with typical designs of the 1920s, might be irritated by 1960s designs. This is likely to become a bigger issue in the future, as design changes accelerated in the late 1960s and 1970s. I shudder to think what might transpire if the psychedelic patterns of this era were recreated – though it may well be that people who lived through that era are more used to dealing with change and will be able to cope with it.

Table 11.1 Dementia 'friendly' features in long-term care residential facilities

Home-like	Consider culture, food, language, religion
Age-appropriate	Consider colour scheme, fittings and furnishings
Lighting	Avoid too bright or too dark, need dim night-lights
Acoustics	No reverberating sound, avoid public address system
Size	6–15 residents in a dementia-specific unit, 20–25 residents if challenging behaviour is not an issue
Security/safety	Unobtrusive safety features (hiding or disguising exit doors), secure doors, electronic tags, avoid overemphasis on safety
Design	Good visual access to most important sections (bedroom, dining room, toilet) from living area. Avoid long corridors, many corners, recessed doors
Floors	Non-slippery, no distracting patterns, no little steps
Toilets/ bathrooms	Good signage, wheelchair access, grab bars
Bedrooms	Single rooms
Living rooms	More than one needed, different sizes, comfortable chairs (not too low), TV, radio, DVD, internet, computer games, magazines, books
Kitchen/dining	Allow both communal and individual meals and possible participation in meal preparation
Outside space	Gardens, paths, seats, security
Activities	Check the social and activity programme, community and caregiver involvement
Staff	Ask about training programme, note involvement of staff with residents and staff attitudes

Designs need to compensate for the cognitive deficits and challenging behaviour of dementia while allowing staff to have good visual access. Lighting should be sufficient to avoid dark areas, but not too bright, which

can lead to problems with glare and shadows. Dim night-lights might minimise nocturnal confusion. Poor acoustics are a problem, especially where you have uncontrolled noise, such as screaming, from residents in the severe stage of dementia. Some facilities still use a public address system for staff communication and this can add to the problem. Materials that absorb sound are important.

The number of persons to be housed in an area is very important. The ideal size of a facility primarily intended for persons with challenging behaviour is 6 to 15 residents. This usually means that it is a self-contained part of a larger facility. If the facility is required for a person who wanders, the doors need to be locked with either combination lock, security swipe card or keyed access. When challenging behaviour is not an issue, 20 to 25 residents can be reasonably looked after in one section. The overall design should be kept as simple as possible – complexes with long corridors with many corners and recessed doors are hard enough for the staff to find their way around let alone the residents! Safety features should be unobtrusive and it is useful for busy exit doors to be disguised or hidden. Walking surfaces need to be even and with no distracting patterns or a tendency to produce glare. Small steps that are difficult to see may be unsafe.

Toilets should be easily accessible, with good signage, and preferably visible from bedrooms, activity, and living areas so that residents have a better chance of avoiding 'accidents'. Bathrooms need standard safety features including grab bars, non-slip tubs and showers with wheelchair access.

There must be quiet areas of various sizes for residents to sit comfortably in varying degrees of privacy. The seating itself should be safe and comfortable. While recliner chairs may have an important role with people with dementia who are unable to ambulate, they can be dangerous as they are difficult to get out of and falls may occur. Dining areas should allow for both communal and individual meals, as some people are more comfortable eating in company and others alone. In smaller facilities, the kitchen can be incorporated into the home-like design and provide the opportunity for residents to participate in meal preparation.

Secure outside space, preferably with well-designed gardens, rest spots, and walking paths is important for exercise and to assist with some challenging behaviour such as restlessness. Flower and herb gardens also provide excellent sensory stimulation. Other features that can make a facility more home-like include pets, indoor plants, encouraging residents

to help with chores, internet access, and policies that encourage open interaction with the local community including visits from schoolchildren, volunteer groups and church groups. It should be ascertained whether the facility accesses formal visitors schemes such as the Commonwealth Government-funded Community Vistors Scheme in Australia that arrange companionship to residents to combat social and cultural isolation in long-term care facilities.

Another factor that impinges upon facility design is the concept of 'ageing in place', which refers to the person with dementia remaining in the one facility until they die. This can be most successfully achieved in a larger facility that has sections with low-level care and others with high-level skilled nursing care. Some dementia facilities, particularly those that cater for challenging behaviours, do not provide care for persons who are bedbound with advanced dementia, and will require the person to be transferred to another section should that eventuality arise.

The downside of creating a home-like atmosphere is that sometimes the design may increase the risk of accidents by incorporating furniture and fittings that are easy to trip over. Falls resulting in hip fractures are a major problem in long-term care facilities. Although hip surgery has improved considerably, it is sobering to realise that about one third of older people with hip fractures die within 12 months.[6]

Certain features, such as pets, may not appeal to all residents and there is always the fear that atypical infections such as scabies might be acquired from a pet. Another problem is that tough (some might say pedantic) regulations may prevent particular resident activities. Meredith Gresham, an occupational therapist, told me of an experience in a residential facility where she encouraged some residents to assist in meal preparation – only to be told that food safety legislation forbade the residents from eating the food due to food hygiene concerns! Obviously there needs to be a balance between creating a safe, hygienic environment backed up by appropriate regulations and the provision of optimal quality of life through a home-like atmosphere.

Types of residential care for dementia

The type of facility that is appropriate for an individual will vary, depending upon the severity of the dementia and degree of behavioural complications. Facilities designed for wanderers need to be secure, with ample space for them to exercise safely both indoors and outdoors.

On the other hand, a person with severe dementia who doesn't wander, or who has limited mobility and no other challenging behaviour, can often be managed in a mainstream facility. Indeed, most long-term care facilities have a large proportion of residents with dementia. Therefore, all facilities need to have design features to assist in dementia care, though such features are extremely variable from one facility to the next.

Each country has its own terminology to describe different types of residential care, and some countries have had changes in their terminology in recent years, thus complicating international comparisons. In general there are two levels of care available: a low-level care that provides meals, accommodation, social activities and limited assistance with medication and activities of daily living, and a high-level care that includes full assistance with activities of daily living (where required) along with skilled nursing care.[7]

While many long-term care facilities specialise in either low-level or high-level care, some cover both. In the US, for example, the type of facility that caters for ageing in place with different levels of care is known as a Continuing Care Retirement Community (CCRC).[8]

The types of facilities that cover low and high-level care needs vary from country to country. In the US, low-level care facilities include the self-funded 'board and care homes' (sometimes known as group homes) that provide help with some activities of daily living, and 'assisted living facilities' that generally provide help with bathing, dressing and toileting, as well as assistance with medications, and facilitate additional services such as attendance at appointments. Assisted living facilities are covered by Medicaid but not Medicare and so for many individuals are also self-funded. High-level care nursing homes or skilled nursing facilities are certified under federal regulations and need to fulfil detailed accreditation standards to be eligible for Medicare and Medicaid reimbursements.[9] Information about the quality ratings of individual nursing homes is available on the Medicare website (see Appendix 2).

In the UK, the low-level care 'residential homes' and the high-level care 'nursing homes' were amalgamated some years ago to become 'care homes'. Approximately 60 per cent of care homes focus on residential care. Fees are paid by a mix of self-funding, pensions, or the NHS with a means-tested system determining what an individual has to pay. The trend in the UK has been for increasing numbers of privately owned care homes with lower numbers of care homes owned by local authorities.[10]

In Canada there are a plethora of terms that cover this field largely because long-term care is the responsibility of the provinces rather than the federal government and there has been an absence of coordinated planning. Unlike other countries, there is a lack of clear distinction about levels of care in the provincially regulated long-term care facilities which receive some level of government funding and have a variety of names including 'nursing homes', 'residential care homes', 'personal care homes' and 'special care homes'. Many Canadians in this level of care reside in unregulated facilities, either 'retirement homes', which are mainly privately owned facilities that provide meals, housekeeping and basic services for a self-funded monthly fee without government requirement to have a minimum level of medical care, or 'assisted living centres', which are mainly self-funded, offering housing and home care services including meals, housekeeping and personal support.[11, 12, 13]

Low-level care (assisted living) long-term care facilities

Low-level care facilities are not specifically intended for persons with dementia but in reality many people with mild to moderate dementia reside in them. Thus a well-designed low-level care facility should have many of the features previously described for dementia. Some will even have locked doors, though this tends to impinge upon the rights of residents who do not have dementia.

In most facilities, individual residents have their own rooms with en suite bathrooms. Most are designed like bed-sitters with a section of the room used as a living area and the rest as a bedroom. Sometimes there is a kitchenette. The size varies between facilities and in some of the older ones the rooms can be quite small. Residents are usually encouraged to use their own furniture from home to assist in the settling-in process, particularly items such as TVs, stereos, sideboards, bookcases, coffee tables, lounge chairs, pictures and mementos. Obviously not much can fit into a room so difficult choices often have to be made.

Professional supervision, where provided, is largely limited to medication administration and in some facilities will attract extra fees. There is minimal health professional involvement from day to day. Personal care assistants might ensure that the residents have their meals, are looking after their personal hygiene and are participating in social activities organised by the facility, although the latter only tends to occur in regulated facilities. Assistance with specific aspects of personal care will be given if required.

As many residents with dementia have some challenging behaviour, there is often a need for the staff to have a plan of behaviour management.

In my experience, most physically fit people with mild to moderate dementia who require residential care are well suited to this type of care. Another group that this type of care might suit is married couples, when the caregiver is too frail to continue care at home. Sometimes adjoining or shared rooms can be arranged.

High-level (nursing home, skilled nursing) long-term care facilities

The majority of residents in these facilities have dementia. Many of the others have milder mental impairments due to strokes, Parkinson's disease, depression and other medical conditions. It is important to realise that most people with dementia do not require dementia-specific facilities as described below. Unless there are particular behavioural concerns that require specific care, standard high-level long-term care facilities are equipped to manage people with dementia.[14]

The main difference between low-level and high-level care is the amount of assistance required for the resident. In general, most persons with severe dementia and many with moderate dementia require high-level care, needing assistance with eating, dressing, bathing, toileting, and often with mobility. Many residents are chairbound or bedbound and require two people to move them, often with the aid of a mechanical lifter. While personal care and nursing assistants can accomplish many of these tasks, there is also a need for registered nurses to be present full time to manage medications, change catheters, apply dressings, administer special feeds and provide overall supervision of the other staff. This will involve regular interactions with the residents' doctors as well as with their families and friends. Other health professionals required in high-level facilities include physiotherapists (particularly to assist with rehabilitation), diversional therapists and music therapists.

Dementia-specific facilities

Dementia-specific facilities include special care dementia units, Alzheimer special care units, psychogeriatric aged care facilities, high dependency units, psychogeriatric extended care units and intensive care residential behavioural units, all of which cater for people with dementia with behavioural disturbances too severe to be managed in standard long-term care facilities.[15, 16] Such behaviours include severe aggression, marked agitation and incessant wandering. In Australia, about 6 per cent of

high-level care facilities are dementia-specific and about 5 per cent of low-level care facilities, for apart from the behavioural disturbance, the person with dementia may still be relatively independent.[17] Historically in most countries this type of care was primarily provided in psychiatric hospitals but over the last 30 years there has been a move away from the mental health sector into the aged care sector with relatively few psychiatric hospitals now being used for this purpose, although there is regional variation within countries in levels of provision available.

Some people might think that any person with a dementia diagnosis should be in a dementia-specific facility. This is unnecessary, as there is no evidence that these types of units are any better than a standard long-term care facility for the average person with dementia. As described earlier, dementia-specific units should be small (catering for between 6 and 15 residents) and self-contained, although usually part of a larger facility. Units of larger size are likely to amplify the behaviours they are intended to deal with. The staff needs to have specific training and expertise in the management of behavioural disturbances. In addition, staff numbers have to be higher than average to ensure that the individual residents get sufficient attention in a safe manner.

In my opinion, dementia-specific facilities should not be viewed as a permanent placement. Most severe behavioural disturbances subside with a combination of good management and time. Thus after 6 to 12 months, most residents have improved sufficiently to be managed in a standard facility. Unfortunately, this doesn't tend to happen, and most dementia-specific facilities have many residents who no longer need to be there – or indeed didn't really need to be there in the first place. This tends to block access to dementia-specific facilities for the persons who really need them, who are then often inappropriately placed in standard facilities where major problems ensue. In some places, such as the state of Victoria in Australia, the local Aged Persons Mental Health Services are involved in managing these facilities and act as gatekeepers. This allows more appropriate use of the resource for the broader community and it is the process favoured by most professional advocates.

The residential care systems in the UK, Canada and the US

While the types of residential care available in the UK, Canada and the US are very similar, the processes required for consumers and carers to access residential care and the funding of care in each country varies considerably.

It is beyond the scope of this book to provide detailed coverage of these issues and so apart from a general overview, more precise details are best obtained from websites that I have listed in Appendix 2.

UK

An assessment of care needs by the local authority social services to determine eligibility for public assistance with residential fees is essential before entry into a care home, whether it be at residential home or nursing home level of care. Once this has been completed, the local authority undertakes a financial assessment of the individual's means-tested ability to pay for their care needs and what, if any, level of contribution they should pay towards their care. Although the process of the financial assessment is the same throughout the UK, the assets test has regional variation of upper and lower limits. Individuals with capital below the lower limit are fully funded by the local authority, while those with capital above the upper limit are liable to pay the full rate.[18]

Care homes are regulated by the Care Quality Commission (CQC) which is also responsible for regulating the quality of care in hospitals and other community and health services. The standards of quality and safety are regularly monitored by CQC inspections that are published on its website.[19]

Canada

Although admission to long-term residential care is based on a needs assessment, the assessment and how it is accessed varies between provinces and territories. In general, nursing homes are regulated and Accreditation Canada has developed long-term care standards. In all jurisdictions, the level of personal contributions is means tested, with government subsidies available to support those who require financial assistance.[20]

Long-term residential care is the responsibility of the provinces and, unlike acute hospitals, is not covered by the Canada Health Act and nor is it fully insured in any of the provinces or territories. It is perhaps a factor contributing to the large number of Canadians, in 2010 estimated as around 7550 on any given day, in an acute hospital awaiting placement to a long-term care or rehabilitation facility. Repeated concerns have been expressed about the accessibility, affordability and quality of long-term care in Canada.[21, 22]

US

No formal needs assessment is required before admission into long-term residential care in the US. Indeed it is left very much in the hands of the older person and their caregiver how much advice they obtain from geriatricians and other specialist aged care clinicians about their options. Approximately 70 per cent of Americans receive funding from Medicaid for their nursing home care, although eligibility is means tested.[23]

Facilities that receive federal funding have to meet accreditation standards which are monitored through regular inspections with results published on the Medicare website. However there are numerous nursing homes that are not accredited.

Concerns about the quality and future of long-term residential care

The quality of care in long-term care facilities has been a controversial area in recent years with a series of incidents being highlighted in the media worldwide. In Australia, for example, several violent incidents in nursing homes prompted the Minister for Ageing to commission a report in 2008 which made a series of recommendations regarding the care of these residents in aged care facilities including the establishment of a Psychogeriatric Care Expert Reference Group, which I chaired, to provide advice on these issues, particularly about models of treatment and care, innovative service delivery, and strategies to improve collaboration between service providers, policy makers and administrators.[24]

It is too simplistic to relate quality of care with the amount of funding available to a facility – some facilities that charge enormous fees and have a very attractive design can provide very poor care. However, a facility having adequate numbers of well-trained and reasonably paid staff with good leadership in a well-designed facility is likely to cost more than the average to run. The cost of having a quality long-term care system that is appropriately regulated and meets the needs of its residents is perhaps more than what is currently in the system in any country.

There are a number of concerns regarding the future of residential long-term care. The baby boomer generation has arrived and apart from the huge population increase that will happen in people aged 65 years and over in the next two decades, there is likely to be a change of expectations about what they will expect from care providers. In addition, many baby boomers have inadequate savings for their long-term care needs.

There is already an undersupply of beds with consequent pressures on caregivers and acute hospitals that are blocked with people awaiting a place.[25] This is accentuated by inadequate governmental and non-governmental investment in long-term care with much more capital investment required for building improvements with greater attention paid to their design.

Worldwide nursing shortages are accentuated in the residential aged care sector which has greater problems in attracting and retaining staff due to the nature of the work and relatively poor (compared to acute hospitals) pay rates. The high staff turnover endemic in many facilities further exacerbates the difficulties in implementing effective training programmes essential to improving dementia care.[26] Special needs groups – residents with severe challenging behaviour; residents under the age of 60 years; and residents from ethnic minorities – are inadequately catered for now and are likely to remain so in the foreseeable future.[27]

Summary

For many reasons, it is a good idea for caregivers to prepare for residential care well before it is needed. This should involve finding out about local facilities and becoming informed about facility features indicative of quality care. There are generally three types of residential long-term care facilities – low-level (assisted living, residential home), high-level (nursing home) and dementia-specific facilities. Only residents with severe behavioural problems need the latter. There a number of concerns about the future direction of residential aged care.

CHAPTER 12

Ethical and Legal Issues

Ethical principles

A number of ethical principles underpin the way we lead our lives. One of the most important of these is *autonomy*, which is the individual's right to be self-governing – in other words, to exercise self-direction, freedom and moral independence. Because dementia fundamentally impairs the capacity of an individual to be autonomous, many ethical and legal problems that arise in dementia care occur around this principle due to conflicts involving decision-making capacity. For example, competency to manage finances, to drive a car, to participate in research, and to decide where to live are common areas of concern discussed later in this chapter.

Other ethical principles that have direct bearing on many of these situations also need to be considered.[1] For caregivers and health professionals, *beneficence*, which means doing good or conferring benefits that enhance personal or social wellbeing, and *non-maleficence*, which means doing no harm, are often the ethical basis of the care being provided. Sometimes these principles may come into conflict and at these times the principle of *justice* may come into play. Justice is about fairness and impartiality and the need to find a balance between competing interests; examples include balancing the desire of the person with dementia to live alone in their own home with the concerns of caregivers about hygiene and safety, and balancing the potential benefits of a drug treatment against the risk of serious side effects. Ultimately, when a person with dementia is found to be incompetent to make a particular decision, it is essential that the needs of the person with dementia, rather than the needs of caregivers, health professionals or others, be the basis of the decision that is arrived at

– in other words, the decision must provide a just outcome for the person with dementia.

Mental competency: decision-making capacity

A fundamental impact of dementia upon an individual is to impair their decision-making capacity and hence their ability to remain autonomous. To have the mental capacity to make a decision, the person must be capable of understanding the nature of the decision and the effects that the decision will have upon the person and others.[2] It is important to understand that mental competence is not 'all or nothing'. For example, a person with dementia may be mentally incompetent to give informed consent for a complex medical procedure but competent to decide whether they wish to give their power of attorney to their spouse. It is crucial in respecting the autonomy of the person with dementia to ensure that they retain their rights to make decisions about things they remain competent to decide upon. A person with dementia whose finances are managed by their guardian, for example, may be able to decide upon where they want to live or what medical treatment they wish to receive. The guardian in these circumstances should not attempt to impose their will upon the person with dementia, although of course they have the right to provide their views on the matter.

How is decision-making capacity determined?

Peteris Darzins from the Monash University in Melbourne and colleagues from Canada have provided lucid practical guidelines for the assessment of mental capacity with 'the six step capacity assessment process'. These guidelines are easy to follow, sensible and fair. Although competency assessments can be made by a variety of health professionals, usually medical specialists, in particular psychiatrists, perform them. It is useful for family caregivers to understand the process as well.[3]

Step 1 – Is there a trigger to make an assessment?
I have often been asked by family caregivers to assess whether their relative is competent to make a will at a time when that relative has no plans to make a will. In these circumstances I suggest they return when there is a plan to make a will, as an assessment is otherwise of little value. In other words, there needs to be a valid trigger for the assessment. There is no need to make any competency assessment without such a trigger.

Valid triggers may include concerns about the person's ability to make financial decisions after bills have been left unpaid or the person with dementia's apparent inability to make appropriate critical decisions about personal or medical care.

Step 2 – Engage the person with dementia in the process

This means that the person with dementia should be adequately informed about the reason for the assessment and efforts made to gain their assent to participate in the process. This step needs to be handled with some delicacy, as many individuals will become indignant and defensive when their competency is questioned. Sometimes caregivers wish to avoid this step on the grounds that the person's mental incompetence is self-evident and they do not want to upset them. While the sentiments are understandable, this approach would deny the person with dementia the right to be properly assessed.

Step 3 – Information gathering

To determine competency, the assessor needs as much information as possible about the situation. This is particularly important with assessments for the capacity to make a will (testamentary capacity), where full knowledge of the person's assets and their natural beneficiaries is needed. However, it is not only information of a factual nature that is required, but also the attitudes, values and goals of the person being assessed. In this area, caregivers can provide valuable information. Cultural and ethnic influences need to be considered as well.

Step 4 – Education

The importance of this step is that the person with dementia is given every opportunity to demonstrate their competence by being provided with adequate information about the situation. Sometimes people with dementia appear to be making incompetent decisions but, when fully informed of the ramifications of the decision they were apparently going to make, change their mind to a decision that is competent. Ignorance should not be allowed to be the basis of a competency decision. Often caregivers are not aware that lack of knowledge lies behind what appears to be stubborn refusal to 'do the right thing'. Nor should reasonable indecision about which medical treatment to follow be the basis of a competency decision. A diagnosis of cancer can lead to prolonged indecision about treatment in

fully competent people so it would not be surprising that a person with dementia might have similar difficulty.

Step 5 – Capacity assessment

In this step, the assessor tests the ability of the person with dementia to make the decision by seeing how well they understand or appreciate the decisions they face. If the person with dementia doesn't understand the ramifications of their decision, or appreciate the effects the decision will have upon others, then they are incompetent to make that particular decision.

Step 6 – Acting on the results of the capacity assessment

The results of the assessment may confirm the competence of the person with dementia to make the decision and this should be conveyed to those who expressed the initial concern. If the person with dementia is found to be incompetent, the capacity assessment will form the basis of the appointment of a substitute decision-maker. Importantly, even if the person with dementia is incompetent to make the decision, they may have views about the issue that need to be taken into account by the appointed substitute decision-maker. For example, the person with dementia may not be competent to decide about whether they should be in a nursing home, but may be able to indicate that they would prefer to live in a certain locality.

Substitute decision-makers

Each jurisdiction has its own legislation that provides the legal basis for the appointment of a substitute decision-maker; while there are some differences around the world the general approach is similar. Thus I explain some of the common terms used in this area.

Is it essential that a substitute decision-maker be appointed? In many circumstances decisions for persons with dementia are made by informal caregivers without any legal appointment but with the obvious blessing of the person with dementia. Often it is the spouse that is in this situation and, providing the couple have joint bank accounts to enable the spouse to access finances and the person with dementia does not overtly object to any decisions made by the spouse, this may suffice. In most jurisdictions, such as in the UK, the closest relative is usually accepted as the person recognised as being able to make such decisions, but in some jurisdictions, such as in the Australian state of New South Wales, the emphasis is

on which person is in the closest caregiving relationship, which may not always be the closest relative. However, particularly for financial management, it is highly recommended that formal legal arrangements are made as described below.[4]

Research into the views of persons with dementia about decision-making in comparison with the views of their caregivers has shown that many caregivers do not have a good understanding of the values of the person with dementia.[5] In addition, over time, caregivers tend to increasingly de-emphasise the importance of the values and preferences of the person with dementia in decision-making.[6] Persons with dementia who report more involvement with decision-making tender to be younger, more educated, female, be less impaired, have a non-spouse caregiver and have a more recent diagnosis.[7] Alzheimer Scotland has produced a good practical guide, 'Dementia: Making Decisions', to assist caregivers with decision-making that takes into account the views of the person with dementia.[8]

Advance health care directives

Sometimes called a 'living will', an advance health care directive is a written statement made by a competent person about what medical treatment they would like to receive when they are no longer competent to make the decision. For a person with dementia, it would be wise to cover end-of-life issues such as resuscitation, tube feeding and intravenous therapy. They are not backed by legislation in all countries but when medical decisions are made for an incompetent person, the views expressed when the person was competent should always be taken into account by the substitute decision-maker. By the same token, an incompetent person with dementia might change their views about what treatment they want and in this situation the substitute decision-maker will have to decide which preference reflects the best interests of the person with dementia. If a competent person wishes to make an advance directive, it is advisable to gain medical and legal advice about the format.[9]

Power of attorney, enduring power of attorney, lasting power of attorney, enduring guardianship

A power of attorney is a legal document by which a mentally competent person authorises someone to make decisions and sign papers on their behalf. However, a power of attorney becomes invalid if a person with

dementia loses their decision-making capacity. For this reason, people with dementia require an enduring power of attorney, a document that contains a statement that the authorisation will continue when they lose their mental capacity. In some jurisdictions, an enduring power of attorney needs to be completed with a 'prescribed person', usually a solicitor, barrister or a clerk of the local court and applies only to financial decision-making and if personal, lifestyle and medical treatment decisions are also to be included, an enduring guardianship is required.

In other jurisdictions enduring power of attorney includes decision-making about health care, personal and lifestyle matters as well when they are no longer able to make these decisions themselves. In the UK in 2007, enduring power of attorney, which only covered property and finances, was replaced by the lasting power of attorney (LPA), which has the options of property and financial affairs LPA, and health and welfare LPA, the latter being the equivalent of enduring guardianship.[10] While these extra powers may assure the person with dementia about who will make the decisions, it does not specifically guarantee the content of the decisions, though some written directives might help guide the decision making (such as with an advance health care directive) and the conditions or limitations the person desires. Some jurisdictions have specific requirements about the format of an enduring power of attorney or guardianship. For example, in the UK, the LPA must be completed on the official LPA form obtained from the government website (www.gov.uk/power-of-attorney) which also provides guidance on the steps required. This includes information about who can be the person nominated as the decision-maker (i.e. the attorney), which in the UK is any competent person aged 18 and over who is not bankrupt. Once the LPA has been completed, it can only be used if it is registered with the Office of the Public Guardian. This costs £130 for each type of LPA and the registration process may take up to 10 weeks.[10] In other jurisdictions, the enduring power of attorney or guardianship may need to be registered if land deals are to be transacted with it. As with advance directives, an enduring power of attorney or guardian may be revoked while the person remains competent and they only come into effect when the person loses their competence.[11, 12]

An enduring power of attorney or guardian is usually a family member or close friend. Where an older person has no one to turn to, or does not want to encumber their family or friends, there are several options available, including the person with dementia's solicitor, accountant, or

the Public Trustee, to act as the enduring power of attorney or guardian and look after their affairs.

Guardianship

When a person with dementia no longer has the capacity to make a decision and no formal arrangements are in place for a substitute decision-maker (for example, an enduring power of attorney), in most circumstances their informal caregiver, usually a spouse or child, is able to make many decisions on their behalf. However, when the person with dementia objects to the lifestyle decision being made, or when financial transactions have to be undertaken using their resources, a legally appointed guardian is required.

Guardianship legislation varies from jurisdiction to jurisdiction but there are many features in common. Usually there are two components – financial management, and personal, lifestyle and medical treatment decisions. In many cases, it is only financial decisions that require the appointment of a legal guardian, for example when a house must be sold to enable nursing home placement. In this situation a guardian would be appointed with powers limited to this area. At other times guardianship will include lifestyle decisions, for example medical consent. Two types of guardians can be appointed – a public guardian, or a family member or friend of the person with dementia. Public guardians are usually only appointed in the absence of family or friends or where there is a serious and unresolvable dispute between family members or friends about the person with dementia. This latter situation includes cases where there has been elder abuse.

The guardianship appointment process can be lengthy, though urgent hearings can be obtained in an emergency, at which an interim guardian can be appointed until the situation is fully investigated – an interim guardian might be appointed where it is suspected that a person with dementia is being defrauded, for example. There are two basic criteria to be met for a guardian to be appointed. First, it is necessary to establish that the person with dementia is unable to make a competent decision due to the effects of their illness. This usually requires two health professional reports to establish the extent of the disability. Second, it is necessary to demonstrate that there is a need to appoint a guardian – in other words, it must be shown that there are decisions to be made which an informal caregiver is legally unable to make. Information is gathered about the situation and a tribunal or judicial hearing is held, which all interested

parties, including the person with dementia, are encouraged to attend. A tribunal usually includes a lawyer, a health professional and a lay person on the panel. If the tribunal or judge determines that a guardian should be appointed, it then determines who the appointed guardian should be and the extent of the guardian's powers. For example, if it is intended that the guardian should have the power to authorise nursing home placement against the person with dementia's will, this must usually be explicitly stated in the guardianship order. If a decision required lies outside of the guardian's appointed powers, this will have to be considered by another sitting of the tribunal or judiciary.[13, 14, 15]

Driving

There is no doubt that dementia adversely affects a person's ability to drive. The unresolved question is at what point the person with dementia should cease to drive. The American Academy of Neurology has recommended that all persons diagnosed with dementia should cease driving;[16] in the state of California, the diagnosing doctor must report a diagnosis of Alzheimer's disease, which usually results in revocation of the driving licence. Given that many persons are being diagnosed with very mild dementia these days, mandatory licence revocation appears harsh, as many of them would still be capable of driving safely.

There are numerous potential consequences of having driving privileges revoked. Loss of independence is the major problem. It may be difficult to find alternative transport, though for many people it may well be cheaper to use taxis than to maintain a car. Taxis may be fine for city dwellers, but in rural settings they are not usually a viable option. There are still many older people who have never obtained their driver's licence; when their spouse is no longer able to drive they can become isolated as well. It is not uncommon in such cases to be asked to allow the person with dementia to keep driving providing the spouse always travel with them. Loss of a driving licence can put stress on other family members who may find themselves providing alternative transport. Driving has long been a symbol of independence and therefore losing the right to drive can be shattering, particularly in an otherwise fit person. Some people become quite depressed, as it often symbolises the decline in function that has been occurring in other ways.

Joe was a 65-year-old retired motor mechanic who had been diagnosed with Alzheimer's disease for a year. Cars had been his life. He fixed them,

drove them, watched the Formula 1 Grand Prix on television and regularly went to car rallies. He was proud of his perfect driving record. Joe's wife, Dianne, had noticed that over the previous six months he seemed less sure of himself while driving. There was nothing too dramatic, just some hesitancy at intersections, uncertainty with new road signs and disorientation in unfamiliar areas. Dianne was usually with him so she was able to help. The situation came to a head, though, when some unexpected roadworks required a detour onto a lane on the other side of the road. Joe was slow to react and after almost collecting the detour sign, he overcorrected onto the other side of the road, narrowly missing the oncoming traffic. Joe seemed unaware of the extent of his near miss but Dianne realised that there was a problem. After seeking advice, she arranged for Joe to have a driving assessment with an occupational therapist at the regional driving assessment centre. Joe was livid that anybody should doubt his ability to drive but agreed to have the test, during which it became clear that he was repeatedly making errors in complex situations. Even he began to see that he was not driving to his former capacity. Although extremely disappointed when told that he had failed, he accepted the decision and handed in his licence. For months afterwards he was morbid and pining to drive.

The research on the effects of dementia upon driving ability has been inconclusive in many ways. One study conducted in 1997 at Washington University in Saint Louis, Missouri, demonstrated that while poor driving performance increases with increased severity of dementia, not all people with dementia were unsafe drivers at a given point in time.[17] A second study found that actual crashes do not necessarily occur more frequently as a result of drivers with dementia compared to elderly drivers without dementia, suggesting that the diagnosis of dementia should not be the only reason for revocation of the driving licence.[18] Indeed, it can be difficult to isolate the effects of dementia from other age-related conditions such as poor eyesight and hearing, arthritis, stroke, cardiorespiratory disorders and medication effects. People over the age of 70 have higher rates of road traffic accidents than younger people per kilometre travelled. However, there is evidence that persons with very mild dementia can have problems in on-road tests in dealing with the complexity of unexpected events and multiple road signs. Perception of signs when driving at speed can also be poor.

Unfortunately, simple cognitive tests do not reliably discriminate between safe and unsafe drivers. Some authorities have claimed that tests of attention, visual memory and visuospatial function might identify unsafe drivers, but this has not been confirmed in large studies. Consequently, the

only reliable way to tell whether a person with early dementia is safe to drive is by the use of an in-car, on-the-road evaluation or other functional test to assess driving skills. One of the dilemmas here is that there seems to be great variability in driving assessments, depending on such factors as the jurisdiction in which they occur and whether they are performed by occupational therapists who specialise in assessing people with dementia or by regular driving assessors from the licensing authority who, it seems, can be extremely lenient in their assessments. This is an area that requires better standards.

It should be remembered that driving is a privilege, not a right. Individuals who have chronic progressive disorders such as dementia are obliged to notify the licensing authority of their condition when they believe it impairs their ability to drive safely. Of course, with a condition such as dementia, self-reporting is a rare occurrence.

I believe that all drivers who are diagnosed with dementia who want to keep driving should undergo a baseline driving assessment in their own car by a driving assessor with expertise in this area, usually an occupational therapist. This should be reviewed every 12 months, or earlier if evidence of impaired driving skills emerges through the onset of repeated minor scrapes, for example, or the concerns of an observer. Some people decide of their own accord to stop driving soon after the diagnosis. Everyone should be given the opportunity to make up their own mind, providing they are still safe on the road. Raising the issue of driving soon after diagnosis enables such a decision to be made with less stress to all. It is important to maintain the person with dementia's autonomy for as long as possible.

Sometimes, no matter how much preparation or planning takes place, the person with dementia refuses to accept that they shouldn't drive, even after failing a driving assessment. Various strategies have been used by caregivers to try to get the message across including disabling the car, arranging for the car to be 'stolen' or sold, getting the local police or other respected authority figure to speak to the person with dementia, and arranging insurance documentation that states the driver is uninsured. Many creative methods have been used; eventually one of them usually works.

Research on people with dementia

One of the tenets of medical research, as espoused in various codes of ethics including the World Medical Assembly's Declaration of Helsinki

and regulations such as those of the Medical Research Council in the UK, is that participants in such research should give their informed consent.[19] Some people with mild dementia, many with moderate dementia and almost all with severe dementia will have lost the capacity to give their informed consent to participate in research. Most research studies involving new drug treatments for Alzheimer's disease insist that the person with dementia is competent to provide informed consent and that the primary caregiver should provide proxy consent as well. Some worries have been expressed that some people may lose their decision-making capacity during the course of a long (often 6 to 12-month) study. Others raise concerns that many participants who appear on the surface to be competent to decide seem to have a very questionable grasp of what is expected of them in the research project when they are examined in greater depth. For example, the person with early dementia keen to participate in a trial of a new Alzheimer drug may understand that there is a 50–50 chance of being given a placebo, but may not fully understand the possible side effects of the new drug, and it is important that the person with dementia and their caregivers are aware of the distinction between standard care and research. It should also be remembered that some new treatments prove to be unsafe when tested in humans, as was discovered with the 'Alzheimer vaccine' trial, described in Chapter 2, which resulted in several deaths. In general, however, this approach to drug trials for dementia drugs is seen by most commentators as being ethically sound.[20]

But there are circumstances where the nature of the treatment being studied almost inevitably involves the recruitment of participants incapable of providing informed consent, such as persons with severe dementia complicated by behavioural disturbances. Is the proxy consent of the spouse or guardian an adequate alternative? Possibly, but while this consent would be adequate for a standard treatments, most guardianship legislation does not allow for research consent. In the UK, the Mental Capacity Act 2005 has clarified and enshrined in law the statutory requirements for when adults who lack the capacity to consent are included in medical research studies. In this situation, it is important that the substitute decision-maker acts in the person with dementia's best interests and not those of any other party. It has been proposed that advance health care directives should include a clause about a person's willingness to participate in research, though one evaluation found that this approach seemed to have a detrimental effect upon study enrolment without discernible benefits in assisting in the decision-making process.[21]

Some authorities strongly argue that under no circumstances should persons unable to provide informed consent be allowed to participate in research. The counterargument runs that this would inevitably mean that people with very impaired decision-making would never have the opportunity to benefit from new treatments that have been appropriately researched. In essence, people with severe dementia would be discriminated against.

Electronic tagging of people with dementia

For a long time, many aged care facilities have placed wristbands that contain an electronic tag on people with dementia who wander. All of the potential exit points of the facility have boundary alarms that are set off when the tagged person goes through them, which then allows the staff to bring the person back before they get lost. The advantages of this system are that locked doors and other restraints are avoided. Some concerns have been expressed about loss of liberties but, providing the tags are used judiciously, most authorities believe that this is not an unreasonable approach.

In the US, electronic tagging has been taken one step further. Silicon chips the size of a grain of rice, which are scanned in much the same way as groceries at a supermarket checkout, are now being injected into the upper backs of people with dementia who live in the community. The chips contain identification, contact and medical information in case the person gets lost. The Alzheimer's Society in the UK and Alzheimer's Australia have indicated that chips capable of being detected by satellite on a global positioning system might be useful in the detection of people with dementia that wander and are missing. Both organisations acknowledge the ethical concerns related to privacy and autonomy and the preference of having prior consent from the person with dementia. Nevertheless, the potential for misuse seems very high.[22]

Placement into residential care against the wishes of the person with dementia

Few people with disabilities are keen to leave their own home and move into residential care. Usually it takes a great deal of soul-searching on the part of the person before they can bring themselves to move. Some will stubbornly refuse; even when it is clear to all around that they are living in unsafe circumstances. If the person is mentally competent, however,

they have the right to live in whatever way they wish providing it doesn't impinge upon the rights of others.

When a person with dementia with impaired decision-making capacity is living alone in an unsafe manner, or with a caregiver who is very stressed, the dilemma arises as to when placement against their will into residential care is justified. If the person with dementia lives alone, caregivers become understandably concerned about the increased risk of harm through accidents, often much to the chagrin of the person with dementia, who resents attempts to impinge on their autonomy. Providing the accident risk doesn't appear to place others at risk of harm, for example by driving a car, I generally encourage family members to allow some risks to be taken in order to respect the person's autonomy.

Ultimately, while community services and caregivers can ensure that the home is kept reasonably clean, that food is provided daily, that the laundry is done, bills paid, appointments kept and social activities provided, it is very difficult to prevent accidents occurring during the inevitable long periods that the person with dementia is unsupervised. The situation is accentuated when the person with dementia does not cooperate with caregivers and community services. When the risk of harm outweighs the benefits of the person enjoying their autonomy, it is time to consider placement. Many people with dementia who are initially adamantly opposed to placement will change their mind and agree to 'give it a go' if given support and encouragement over some months to consider other options. Others will remain stubbornly opposed and, as concerns about safety mount, a guardianship order is usually required to authorise placement against the person's will. In my experience, such applications need to be able to demonstrate that a reasonable package of community care has been trialled unsuccessfully before a guardianship order authorises such placement.

When the person with dementia is living with a caregiver, the same principles apply, but the rights of the caregiver also have to be considered. If the person with dementia has a severe behaviour disturbance, for example, exhibiting aggression towards the caregiver, it is understandable that the caregiver may get to the point where they are no longer able to tolerate it. Of course, every effort should be made to treat the aggressive behaviour and provide the caregiver some respite. Often the caregiver has been tolerating the behaviour for a long time before seeking help. Where the person with dementia would be unable to cope in the absence

of the caregiver, and the caregiver is at the end of their tether, it is time for placement.

End-of-life decisions

Unlike the situation with cancer and other terminal illnesses, planning end-of-life decisions has not often been a routine part of dementia care. This is probably due to the difficulty of discussing such issues with a cognitively impaired person and in part to the failure to conceptualise dementia as a terminal illness. Now that early diagnosis is the rule rather than the exception, however, end-of-life decisions can be broached with the person with dementia and their family in the form of advanced health care directives as described earlier in the chapter.[23] Nevertheless, many older people are not very comfortable with this approach.

In the absence of an advanced health care directive from the person with dementia, a good time for substitute decision-makers to discuss end-of-life decisions with medical and nursing staff is at the time of placement into an aged care facility, or possibly during the course of a hospital admission for an intercurrent illness. Issues that should be covered include resuscitation, use of intravenous therapy, and tube feeding. In the absence of a 'Do Not Resuscitate' (DNR) order, staff in hospitals in particular but also in aged care facilities are obliged to commence resuscitation; once that process has commenced, it can be difficult to know when to stop. A DNR order prevents unwanted interventions when prolongation of life is not desired.[24]

Most people with severe dementia become impaired in their ability to eat. Weight loss is common but it is not always due to inadequate diet; it seems to be part of the dementing process. Caregivers become concerned that the person with dementia may 'starve to death' and want to do everything possible to prevent that. What appears to be food refusal often turns out to be an impairment of the ability of the person with dementia to masticate and swallow. A swallowing assessment from a speech pathologist is a good initial step to determine the nature of the problem.

Tube feeding is often mentioned as a possible solution. The tube is administered through a technique known as percutaneous endoscopic gastrostomy (PEG), in which a feeding tube is passed through the abdominal wall and directly into the stomach. Most authorities believe that tube feeding should not be used to treat dementia-related swallowing difficulties. There is no evidence that tube feeding prevents aspiration

of food into the lungs of people with dementia (a common problem in these situations), or increases comfort, weight, quality of life or lifespan. There is evidence that tube feeding results in reduced pleasure from eating, increased use of restraints to prevent the person with dementia from removing the tube, and loss of human contact at meal times.[25]

As far as possible, assisted oral feeding is a better approach, though often time consuming. Many family caregivers visit their relative daily to feed them; this has the added benefit of providing emotional contact. There comes a time when the dementia is so severe that the person with dementia is unable to receive food and water by mouth. It is regarded as ethically permissible to withhold hydration and nutrition in this situation.

Many people with dementia die of pneumonia, often related to their immobility, swallowing problems and reduced resistance to infections. Pneumonia can usually be successfully treated with antibiotics and the first or second bout in a nursing home resident is usually treated routinely though often with a perceptible decline in function after each bout. There often comes the point after several bouts of pneumonia when the family, doctor or nurses question whether further antibiotic therapy is warranted. There is no easy answer to this and decisions need to be individually determined by family consultation with the health professionals involved.

Summary

Many ethical and legal problems that arise in dementia care occur around the principle of autonomy due to conflicts involving decision-making capacity, which becomes impaired by the dementia. The appointment of an enduring power of attorney or guardian allied with an advanced health care directive during early dementia can avoid many later problems. To have the mental capacity to make a decision, the person must be capable of understanding the nature of the decision and the effects that the decision will have upon the person and others. A capacity assessment may be required but should only be undertaken with a valid trigger such as concern about financial mismanagement or the need for placement into an aged care facility. If the person with dementia is found to be incompetent to make the decision, a substitute decision-maker should be appointed. Driving assessments should also be undertaken after diagnosis and repeated at least every six months to determine competence to drive. Other ethical issues that commonly occur include end-of-life decisions such as tube feeding.

The Future

These are exciting times in the field of dementia care. Scarcely a week goes by without the publication of new research findings that provide a better understanding of some aspect of the early diagnosis, potential treatment or prevention of Alzheimer's disease and other dementias. We are on the cusp of being able to reliably identify people before they develop symptoms of dementia and, more importantly, being able to provide interventions that will significantly reduce or eliminate their risk of developing dementia. Just how far away this is and how effective the interventions may be are matters of speculation. In this chapter I provide some educated guesswork about these issues with the assistance of some internationally recognised dementia specialists. Email surveys were sent to Henry Brodaty, Scientia Professor of Ageing and Mental Health, and Perminder Sachdev, Scientia Professor of Neuropsychiatry, both from the University of New South Wales in Sydney; David Ames, Professor of Ageing and Health, Colin Masters, Professor of Pathology, and Michael Woodward, Associate Professor of Geriatric Medicine, each from the University of Melbourne; Gary Small, Professor of Psychiatry and Biobehavioral Sciences, David Geffen School of Medicine at UCLA; and Brian Lawlor, Professor of Psychiatry for the Elderly, Trinity College, Dublin.

Detection of pre-symptomatic individuals and early diagnosis of dementia

Most experts agree that the accurate detection of individuals with pre-symptomatic dementia is an essential prerequisite to the prevention and successful treatment of various types of dementia, especially Alzheimer's disease. There are a number of ways that this could be achieved including diagnostic tests of blood, urine or cerebrospinal fluid (CSF), through

various types of brain scans, and through other tests of brain function. It is likely that a combination of approaches might be necessary to achieve sufficient diagnostic accuracy.

These days most people are used to their doctor ordering blood and urine tests that assist in the diagnosis of their medical condition. Some of these tests are diagnostic of specific illnesses like HIV infection, vitamin B_{12} deficiency or hepatitis C, though most indicate only a general abnormality that could be due to a range of conditions. In many conditions, the precise diagnosis requires a biopsy of the tissue concerned to allow it to be viewed by a pathologist under a microscope. This is usually obtained during a procedure that is designed to be as non-invasive as possible. Most organs of the body are now reasonably accessible for biopsy, either by needle (e.g. breast, liver); endoscope, which is a tube introduced through a body orifice (the bowel in a colonoscopy, the stomach in a gastroscopy); or by keyhole surgery (e.g. ovaries). Brain biopsies require major surgery and it seems unlikely that any advances in the foreseeable future will allow the safe, reliable biopsy of brain tissue from the desired areas of the brain to allow an accurate diagnosis of dementia during life.

Therefore, a considerable amount of research is underway in attempts to find 'biomarkers' for Alzheimer's disease and other dementias. Biomarkers are molecular and biochemical indicators of a disease that can be detected in the blood, urine or CSF of a person with the disease but not in persons without the disease – in other words, they are a diagnostic test.[1, 2] For Alzheimer's disease, an ideal biomarker would be able to detect a fundamental feature of Alzheimer's neuropathology at an early, preferably pre-symptomatic, phase of the illness, in a manner that would reliably allow Alzheimer cases to be distinguished from other types of dementia as well as from persons without dementia. Such a test needs to be simple, inexpensive and non-invasive. In today's terms this would mean a blood or urine test rather than a test of CSF though some new types of brain scan may offer an alternative approach. It is generally accepted that no biomarker is likely to be 100 per cent accurate.[3, 4]

Diagnostic blood tests

Efforts to identify diagnostic biomarkers for Alzheimer's from blood tests have been thwarted by a lack of diagnostic accuracy of candidate markers and the unreliability of testing procedures between laboratories. The best studied biomarker is beta-amyloid protein and the fundamental problem is the uncertainty about whether changes found in blood tests reflect

changes that are happening in the brain. There are increasing doubts about whether blood tests alone will be sufficient for accurate diagnosis.[5]

Undoubtedly many new blood tests are on the horizon and will be touted by their commercial backers as *the* 'Alzheimer's test'. The concern is that none will be sufficiently accurate or reliable, and that many people, including doctors, may be misled and thus make inappropriate diagnoses, which could cause considerable anxiety in the general public. Henry Brodaty, Perminder Sachdev and David Ames each stated that there would not be a single blood test but rather a combination of blood proteins available by around 2020 (personal communication). It was felt that blood tests alone would be unlikely to have sufficient accuracy to be useful.

On the other hand, while blood tests may not be sufficiently reliable to distinguish Alzheimer's disease from other dementias or from normality, they may be useful tests to monitor the progress of the condition and could be used to confirm whether new drug treatments are working.

Diagnostic CSF examination

CSF surrounds the central nervous system (CNS) (brain and spinal cord) cushioning it from shocks; it circulates the CNS and has an important role in its homeostasis and metabolism. Changes that occur in brain structure or function due to disease can be detected by analysis of the CSF, which is usually obtained by needle aspiration from a lumbar puncture (spinal tap). As described in Chapter 6, currently the main reason to examine CSF in dementia assessment is to exclude infections in the CNS and this is infrequently required.

In the hunt for biomarkers for Alzheimer's disease, it is apparent that the accuracy and reliability of candidate protein levels obtained from the CSF is much better than those detected in blood tests. One major protein that has been examined is beta-amyloid protein, which is the main component of the plaques, primarily with a length of 42 amino acids ($A\beta42$). Around 20 studies have now shown that there is about a 50 per cent reduction of $A\beta42$ in the CSF of Alzheimer patients compared with age-matched normal controls, with diagnostic sensitivity and specificity levels ranging between 80 and 90 per cent. However, when compared with other types of dementia the specificity levels drop to around 60 per cent. It is possible that the diurnal fluctuations of $A\beta42$ levels in the CSF interfere with test accuracy.[6, 7]

The other major protein that has been investigated is tau protein found in the microtubules of neurons. Total tau protein in Alzheimer's disease is

increased by approximately 300 per cent compared with normal controls, with diagnostic sensitivity and specificity levels ranging between 80 and 90 per cent. There is age-related variation in total tau protein levels that affects test interpretation.[8, 9]

The major difficulties that affect the interpretation of Aβ42 and total tau levels is that both are altered in people with mild cognitive impairment, not all of whom progress to dementia, and there is poor discrimination between Alzheimer's disease and other types of dementia, even when the tests are used in combination.

A third biomarker, hyperphosphorylated tau protein (p-tau), has been consistently found to be elevated in the CSF of Alzheimer patients. There are around 30 subtypes of p-tau and differences observed in these subtypes are showing promise in distinguishing Alzheimer's disease from other types of dementia including frontotemporal dementia. In addition, p-tau levels in patients with mild cognitive impairment have been found to be predictive of conversion to Alzheimer's disease. Using a combination of Aβ42, total tau and p-tau levels, a Swedish study found that Alzheimer's disease was able to be predicted in mild cognitive impairment patients with 95 per cent sensitivity and 85 per cent specificity. Single assay methods (that require a lower amount of CSF) are currently being investigated in US and European dementia networks and these are likely to be available in a few years.[10, 11]

These promising developments suggest that CSF examination might become a routine component of dementia assessment in order to identify people with mild cognitive impairment at high risk of developing Alzheimer's disease and to assist in differentiating dementia types. As pointed out by Perminder Sachdev, their uptake by clinicians may depend upon the availability of disease-modifying treatments. Such specific treatments will warrant more precise diagnoses and clinicians and patients will be more willing to perform lumbar punctures (personal communication).

Brain scans

Many dementia experts including Gary Small and Michael Woodward believe that neuroimaging – the visualisation of brain structure or function by various scanning techniques – will be a fruitful avenue for early diagnosis (personal communication). The Alzheimer's Disease Neuroimaging Initiative 2 (ADNI 2) is one of the studies funded through the research programme announced by the US National Institutes of Health in 2012.

It aims to examine how brain imaging and other biomarkers can be used to measure the progression of MCI and early Alzheimer's disease.[12] There are many different types of brain scans but basically they examine either brain structure or function.

STRUCTURAL NEUROIMAGING
Routinely available CT and MRI scans provide images of brain structure and, as described in Chapter 6, are very helpful in assisting with diagnosis; as stand-alone tests, however, they cannot provide a dementia diagnosis. Efforts are now underway to create computerised brain atlases of various diseases that might allow a single CT or MRI scan to be compared with known patterns of disease abnormality. Thus, a brain scan of a person with mild memory problems might be consistent with a scan of early Alzheimer's disease or normal ageing. Although this would be helpful, the analysis of changes over time is more important. Currently, serial CT or MRI scans over a period of a year or two can detect progressive atrophy or increasing vascular lesions, but they need to be interpreted in conjunction with the 'gold standard' clinical examination. Volumetric analysis of the hippocampal formation is the best established structural biomarker for Alzheimer's disease, being able to predict conversion from mild cognitive impairment to dementia with about 80 per cent accuracy. In Alzheimer's disease, hippocampal atrophy occurs at a rate of 3 to 7 per cent per annum in comparison with less than 1 per cent per annum in normal controls. Automated procedures to measure hippocampal volume promise to reduce measurement time from two hours to 30 minutes.[13]

It is proposed that dynamic (4-D) brain maps will evolve with the design of mathematical systems to track anatomical changes over time and map dynamic patterns of brain degeneration associated with different illnesses. One of the main advantages of such approaches over the methods described below is that CT and, to a lesser extent, MRI scans are reasonably accessible, affordable, safe and tolerable for older people and will remain necessary to exclude other causes of dementia.

FUNCTIONAL NEUROIMAGING
Dementia is a clinical syndrome defined by brain function, so it is not surprising that scans of brain function are felt by many researchers to hold out the greatest promise for early, reliable diagnosis. Various types of brain scans that measure aspects of brain function have been available for some years, but for the most part have not achieved sufficient accuracy or

reliability to be used other than as a research tool. This is rapidly changing but has yet to be fully achieved.

Positron Emission Tomography (PET) scans involve the measurement of brain glucose metabolism as a marker of brain function by measuring the uptake of a form of radioactive glucose (fludeoxyglucose – FDG) in various parts of the brain. FDG-PET studies have shown reduced activity in the parietal, temporal and prefrontal lobes of the brain in Alzheimer patients and in the frontal and temporal brain regions in persons with frontotemporal dementia. There are similar but less pronounced abnormalities present in people with mild cognitive impairment and conversion to Alzheimer's disease can be predicted with 80 per cent accuracy.[14]

There has also been research that has targeted individuals at high risk of Alzheimer's disease. PET studies in middle-aged persons with the ε4 allele of the APOE gene but no dementia have shown a similar pattern of changes to those found in persons with Alzheimer's disease, implying that they are already showing possible early changes of brain function. More subtle abnormalities of brain function can be detected by comparing scans taken at mental rest and during a brain activation task.

One particularly exciting development has been the ability to detect amyloid plaques, thus measuring the fundamental neuropathological abnormality of Alzheimer's disease. The most extensively studied radiotracer is Pittsburgh compound B (PiB), which attaches to the amyloid plaques. Studies to date confirm high rates of PiB uptake in persons with Alzheimer's disease. Individuals with mild cognitive impairment that have high rates of PiB uptake are at increased risk of converting to Alzheimer's disease. There is still insufficient long-term information available regarding the accuracy of the PiB PET scan as there are a significant minority of normal controls who have positive scans. It is unclear whether these individuals have pre-symptomatic Alzheimer's disease or are false positives.[15] David Ames, Michael Woodward and Perminder Sachdev felt that by 2020 amyloid scanning would be available for clinicians in many specialist centres (personal communication).

PET scans have a number of disadvantages, however. They involve the use of radioactive isotopes, albeit in small amounts, which requires access to a cyclotron, and there are very few PET scans available. While the number of PET scan centres is increasing, they are not going to be routinely available to the general public, although most teaching hospitals will have access to them. PET scans are also reasonably time consuming to perform, require a relatively cooperative subject and are expensive. For all

these reasons, I doubt whether PET scans will have a major impact in the routine detection and management of dementia in the next 20 years, especially as there are other promising alternatives. It is more likely to be used where there is diagnostic uncertainty such as in a younger person with mild cognitive impairment and depression or in assisting with the differentiation of frontotemporal dementia and dementia with Lewy bodies from Alzheimer's disease.

Functional MRI (fMRI) scanning is one alternative to the PET scan. This technique allows the study of brain function and structure simultaneously without exposure to radiation and in less time than PET scanning. Studies have shown that middle-aged persons at high risk of Alzheimer's disease due to carrying the ε4 allele of the APOE gene have different patterns of activation in the areas of the brain affected by Alzheimer's disease during a memory activation task than individuals not carrying the ε4 allele. These changes also predicted decline in memory function over two years. The current direction being taken with fMRI scans is the investigation of changes in functional connectivity between regions of brain activation in normal controls, those with mild cognitive impairment and those with Alzheimer's disease. There is evidence from small studies that changes in functional connectivity precede differences in brain activation in mild cognitive impairment raising the prospect of a pre-symptomatic marker.[16]

As fMRI is a newer technique than PET scanning, much more data will be required before its potential usefulness in routine clinical practice can be determined. It seems promising in the investigation of pre-symptomatic individuals at high genetic risk and will be potentially more accessible than PET scanning. Recent reports of a related fMRI technique, arterial spin labelling MRI that measures blood flow changes in the brain, suggest that it has similar diagnostic accuracy to FDG-PET but is cheaper and without harmful radiation.[17]

Magnetic Resonance Spectroscopy (MRS) makes it possible to examine biochemical changes in the brain and relate them to behaviour and function. As drug treatments for dementia are primarily aimed at altering levels of neurotransmitters in the brain, the biochemical changes detectable by this technique could become a measure of treatment effect. It is debatable at this stage whether MRS will be clinically useful for diagnostic purposes.[18]

Brain function – cognitive tests

Many of the tests of cognitive function now available – both brief screening tests and more detailed neuropsychological tests – have been shown to be predictive of future cognitive decline in persons with mild cognitive changes, but not to the extent that an accurate diagnosis can be made without serial testing. Brief cognitive tests are not very suitable for serial testing of mild impairment, while repeated full neuropsychological assessments are time consuming, expensive and impractical if considered on a large scale. Current research is seeking to identify which neuropsychological tests are most predictive of cognitive decline. In this regard, tests that distinguish failure of information storage and new memory creation from attentional disorders are important for identifying early Alzheimer's disease. This can be achieved by tests that can identify low performance of total recall in spite of efforts by the tester to facilitate recall by cueing, thus indicating poor storage of information. This type of amnestic syndrome 'of the hippocampal type' can identify prodromal Alzheimer's disease in patients with MCI with a sensitivity of around 80 per cent and a specificity of around 90 per cent. It should be noted that this only applies to Alzheimer's disease and not other types of dementia where prediction is much less accurate.

A possible alternative, developed in Australia by David Darby, a behavioural neurologist from Victoria, is CogState, a computer-based test designed to measure cognitive performance in about 15 to 18 minutes. It is available over the internet. CogState measures objective speed and accuracy in a card game format, which minimises issues related to culture or language. Individual test results have little meaning unless significantly abnormal. It has been designed specifically for multiple testing, as the intended use is to monitor the progress of individuals over time by comparing later test results with their baseline tests. Any significant declines over time are highlighted and recommendations made for a full medical review.[19]

There are a number of concerns with this and other similar tests. It remains unproven whether the detection of decline in cognitive function by this technique is an accurate predictor of dementia, although research is currently being undertaken to examine this. It also targets the 'worried well' that are searching for reassurance, which may or may not be provided. As any change detected would then require a full medical evaluation to determine the cause and its significance, it is likely that in many cases diagnostic uncertainty will remain and further full medical evaluation 12 or more months down the track will be required.

Neuropsychological testing will remain a key component of early identification of people with dementia but its widespread use is limited by availability of trained neuropsychologists, cost, the time required for testing (two or three hours of testing, and another two or three hours of analysis and report writing), and validity in people from a non-English speaking background.

Overall, it seems that in the foreseeable future early diagnosis will involve the monitoring of high-risk individuals – for example, those with genetic risk factors, multiple vascular risk factors or with mild cognitive changes – from after the age of 50 years, and lower-risk individuals from the age of 70 or 75 years. Monitoring may involve a screen of CSF and/or blood tests to detect biomarkers of Alzheimer's disease, serial brain scans and serial tests of cognitive function. A combination of these tests may indicate the likelihood that the individual has pre-symptomatic or mildly symptomatic dementia, especially Alzheimer's disease. Such findings will only be useful if effective preventive and treatment strategies are available. This approach is consistent with the new diagnostic criteria for Alzheimer's disease that were released in 2011 and are discussed in more detail later in the chapter.[20]

Brain function – smell tests

A number of studies have shown that smell perception changes in the very early stages of Alzheimer's disease. Research examining whether odour identification tests could be used to predict the development of Alzheimer's disease in normal individuals or those with MCI are inconclusive and there is insufficient evidence to promote their use at present. There might be a role for such tests in a broadly based screening strategy if large-scale prospective longitudinal studies demonstrate that they are reliable enough to warrant use, as they will be relatively inexpensive, brief and non-invasive.[21]

New diagnostic criteria for Alzheimer's disease and dementia

New diagnostic criteria for Alzheimer's disease were released by the National Institute on Aging and the Alzheimer's Association in the US in 2011. They are based on specific neuropsychological and clinical features in combination with presence of one or more of the following: medial temporal lobe atrophy on MRI scan; abnormal CSF biomarkers; specific

functioning on PET scan; or the presence of a proven Alzheimer's disease autosomal dominant mutation within the immediate family. They provide a platform for research to refine the previously described biomarkers and for early intervention strategies for individuals who are at high risk of developing Alzheimer's disease at a time when they are either pre-symptomatic or have minimal symptoms.[22, 23]

The American Psychiatric Association's fifth version of the *Diagnostic and Statistical Manual of Mental Disorders (DSM-5)* will be released in 2013. A new category of 'Neurocognitive Disorders' has been devised to include current diagnostic categories such as dementia, mild cognitive disorders and amnestic syndromes. Neurocognitive disorders are subdivided into 'major neurocognitive disorders' and 'minor neurocognitive disorders'; the term 'dementia' has been eliminated with the change primarily driven by the view that the word dementia is stigmatising, particularly for younger people with HIV-associated dementia.[24]

In *DSM-5* the term major neurocognitive disorder essentially replaces the term dementia – but they are not equivalent. In *DSM-5* there is an emphasis on decline from previous level of functioning rather than deficits with definitions largely based on neuropsychological test parameters (two or more standard deviations below appropriate norms). While dementia has required evidence of impairment in two or more cognitive domains, one of which has to be memory, major neurocognitive disorder requires substantial decline in only one cognitive domain and it does not have to be memory. Minor neurocognitive disorder is characterised by modest cognitive decline typically involving performance one to two standard deviations below appropriate norms and insufficient to interfere with independence. This is the category in which MCI will sit, although it is another term that has been eliminated.[25]

It is too early to know what impact these changes will have in the US (the primary audience for *DSM-5*) and elsewhere around the world. More people will be diagnosed with major neurocognitive disorder than we are used to seeing with dementia because only one cognitive domain has to be affected and it does not need to be memory. It is important to stress that the previously mentioned new diagnostic criteria for Alzheimer's disease still require there to be two cognitive domains of impairment before dementia is diagnosed so there is, in effect, likely to be three tiers of diagnosis occurring, with dementia unofficially sitting within the major neurocognitive disorder category as a more severe version. This is likely to be very confusing for clinicians let alone patients.[26]

Work is currently under way on the next version of the World Health Organization's *International Classification of Diseases (ICD)*. This version, *ICD-11*, is due for release in 2015 and one of the challenges will be to harmonise it with *DSM-5* and the new Alzheimer's disease criteria.

Prevention of dementia

As described in Chapters 2 and 3, multiple risk factors for Alzheimer's disease and vascular dementia have now been identified, so theoretically it should be possible to prevent dementia. In 2002, when I surveyed international dementia experts about when it might be possible to prevent dementia for the first edition of this book (then titled *Dealing with Dementia*), the consensus was that this might happen in the next ten years. In the case of Alzheimer's disease, there was general agreement that interventions that prevent amyloid plaque formation will be the cornerstone of therapy, and that the agents involved will also be used to treat symptomatic Alzheimer's disease. The extent to which attention to vascular risk factors such as control of hypertension, cessation of smoking, obesity, and the use of statin medication, may reduce dementia risk remain unclear. In 2002, Brian Lawlor and Michael Woodward felt that delay in the onset of Alzheimer's disease might be reasonably achieved by attention to vascular risk factors alone but their hopes that this would become clearer by now have not eventuated (personal communication). Colin Masters felt that vascular dementia could theoretically be completely prevented by targeting vascular risk factors but this also remains uncertain (personal communication).

Research over the last ten years has been inconclusive about the most effective strategies and the timing of interventions, particularly regarding control of hypertension. In 2012 the dementia experts were more circumspect about prevention. Michael Woodward stressed that public health approaches based on the previously mentioned strategies were the most likely to work for Alzheimer's disease and vascular dementia, but the challenge was to get sufficient evidence that will increase acceptance and uptake by the general public. Henry Brodaty agreed with this and noted that this approach would only delay dementia onset. David Ames and Gary Small felt that a beta-amyloid vaccination approach mightbe possible, perhaps in combination with other therapies, but David Ames felt it wouldn't be available until around 2030. Henry Brodaty felt that vaccines would only be available for high-risk individuals (personal communication).

One of the main challenges facing this field is to obtain sufficient evidence about different interventions to determine their effectiveness in dementia prevention, whether by delay or by eradication. It will take many years of field testing to evaluate their degree of effectiveness and the relative merits of different interventions and combinations of interventions. This is at least partially due to the fact that interventions need to be applied some decades before disease onset, in midlife at least, as risk factors such as low education, hypertension, diabetes, hyperlipidaemia, obesity and diabetes appear to exert their effect mainly in this period. Despite the wide range of dementia risk factors identified in recent years, the main hopes of Alzheimer's disease prevention rest in the development of new drugs that target the accumulation of amyloid. In other words, attention to the other risk factors alone may have only limited benefit by delaying onset of disease.

Treatment of dementia

More effective disease-modifying treatments for symptomatic Alzheimer's disease will prevent amyloid plaque formation by interfering with the amyloid cascade. A number of other types of treatments could also work. Two exciting treatments that may ultimately become important components of therapy are gene therapy and foetal stem cell grafts. The potential is enormous, though there are many scientific, ethical and logistical hurdles to jump before they can be used. If a 'cure' for Alzheimer's disease and other degenerative dementias is ever developed, it is likely to involve one of these therapies, but it may well be at least 20, if not 50, years away. In recent years a large number of Phase III trials, the stage of drug development where efficacy is determined, have had disappointing results including promising drugs such as latrepirdine (Dimebon) that had two large negative trials leading to the discontinuation of the drug's development in 2012.[27] However there are numerous drugs in Phase II studies that hold out hope for new therapies in the next five to ten years.

Secretase inhibitors

Secretase inhibitors work by inhibiting or modulating one of two enzymes – gamma secretase or beta secretase which are involved in the production of beta-amyloid protein.[28, 29] A decade ago there was much optimism that secretase inhibitors would be the next major advance in the treatment of

Alzheimer's disease but subsequent multicentre controlled trials involving gamma secretase inhibitors have yielded disappointing results.

Tarenflurbil was the first gamma-secretase modulator to reach the final stage of clinical development. Surprisingly, Phase III trials demonstrated no clinical benefit with the speculative explanation being that there was inadequate CNS penetration. Phase III trials of a second gamma-secretase inhibitor, Semagacestat, were stopped in 2011 when preliminary results showed that it did not slow disease progression and had toxic effects, with worsening of clinical measures of cognition and the ability to perform activities of daily living. This toxicity was felt to be due to its inhibition of Notch cleavage, a receptor found in the cell membrane.[30, 31]

It is now felt that selective gamma-secretase inhibitors which have better brain penetrance and spare the Notch receptor might be more effective and tolerable. Another gamma-secretase inhibitor Avagacestat completed Phase 1 studies successfully in 2011.[32]

Trials involving beta-secretase inhibitors are not as far advanced. In December 2012, Merck announced that it had begun enrolling for the largest clinical trial of a β-secretase (BACE1) inhibitor in Alzheimer's disease patients. Initially, the Phase II study of MK-8931 will enrol 200 subjects with mild to moderate Alzheimer's disease, due for completion in late 2013, and if this is successful Merck will enrol 1800 subjects in an 18-month Phase III study due for completion in 2016.[33] There are also plans for a study of prodromal Alzheimer's disease. Meanwhile Eli Lilly and Company have a Phase II trial under way with the β-site amyloid protein cleaving enzyme (BACE) inhibitor LY2886721 in patients with MCI and positive PiB scans which is due for completion in 2014.[34]

Although the Merck study of MK-8931 involves mild to moderate Alzheimer's disease, there is a view that secretase inhibitors might only be effective in pre-symptomatic Alzheimer's disease or mild cognitive impairment due to Alzheimer's disease. It may well be that once the level of damage reaches the extent that dementia has occurred, stopping the further accumulation and removal of beta-amyloid protein might not improve cognition.

Beta-amyloid vaccination

Immunisation (vaccination) aims to increase the cleavage (breakdown) of beta-amyloid protein. There are a number of approaches that involve the production of antibodies, with active vaccinations having a higher risk

of adverse effects than passive vaccinations. In 2012 studies involving two compounds, bapineuzumab and solanezumab, were completed with disappointing results.[35, 36] Vanutide cridificar, an active vaccination, is in Phase II trials that are due for completion in 2013 while a second active immunotherapy compound CAD106 was reported in 2012 to be safe with an acceptable antibody response in a Phase I study from Sweden.[37]

Two Phase III studies of intravenous bapineuzumab in mild to moderate Alzheimer's disease showed no improvement in cognition or function, despite lowering beta-amyloid levels in the brain.[38, 39] This resulted in the sponsors, Pfizer and Janssen Alzheimer Immunotherapy, having to discontinue the bapineuzumab research programme in August 2012. Similarly two Phase III studies of solanezumab in mild to moderate Alzheimer's disease showed no improvement in cognition or function, although there was evidence of slowing of cognitive decline in subjects with mild Alzheimer's disease by 34 per cent and they showed a reduction in CSF beta-amyloid.[40, 41] There are further studies in progress with solanezumab.

In October 2012, the Dominantly Inherited Alzheimer Network (DIAN) announced that they had chosen solanezumab and gantenerumab for clinical trials that will commence worldwide in 2013 to try to prevent dementia in people who are on the path to Alzheimer's disease due to an inherited autosomal-dominant mutation.[42]

If effective, these treatments are likely to be used in combination with other therapies, some of which are currently available but are unproven such as statins, anti-inflammatory drugs, control of blood pressure in midlife, antioxidants, and folic acid, along with lifestyle changes with diet (low in fat; high in grains, greens and fish), optimal alcohol consumption, physical and mental exercise, avoidance of head injuries, and no smoking. These treatments are also likely to be beneficial for vascular dementia, mixed vascular/Alzheimer dementia and dementia with Lewy bodies, though the degree of benefit is uncertain.

Gene therapy

In 2001, the first study to test the safety of gene therapy in Alzheimer's disease with the drug CERE-110 was commenced in San Diego and involved eight patients with mild Alzheimer's disease. Promising Phase I study results were published in 2005 and currently a Phase II trial involving 50 patients is underway.[43]

In gene therapy, fibroblast cells obtained from the skin of the patients are cultured and then genetically modified in a test tube to produce and secrete the human nerve growth factor (NGF) molecule. The patients receive intracerebral injections of their own fibroblasts into the regions of their brains where neurons are undergoing atrophy as a result of Alzheimer's disease. The eventual goal is to determine whether NGF produced by the cells implanted into the brain can prevent the death of some nerve cells affected by the Alzheimer's disease, and enhance the function of some remaining brain cells. If successful, gene therapy may be used in the future in combination with drugs that prevent amyloid plaque formation. The drugs will stop further damage from occurring while the gene therapy will attempt to restore neurons that have already perished.

Stem cell grafts

This is a very controversial topic, as evidenced by the impassioned debates that took place in the Australian Parliament about the use of foetal stem cells before legislation was passed in December 2002. A stem cell is an unspecialised cell that has the ability to renew itself indefinitely. Under appropriate conditions it can give rise to a wide range of mature cell types in the human body. Any disorder that involves loss of or injury to normal cells is a candidate for stem cell therapy. In this regard, many disorders of the nervous system, including Alzheimer's disease, Parkinson's disease and the other degenerative dementias, are prime targets for neuronal stem cell therapy.

Stem cells can be obtained from a variety of sources including embryos, foetal tissue and some adult tissues. Until recently, adult neurogenesis (nerve cell formation) was not thought to be possible, hence the debate over the use of foetal stem cells. It is now known that adult neurogenesis may be active in the human brain as a response to Alzheimer's disease so adult stem cell therapy may be possible. In July 2012, the Alzheimer's Society in the UK announced that it would only fund stem cell research that involved either adult stem cells or induced pluripotent stem cells as these do not have the same ethical concerns as embryonic and foetal stem cells.[44]

How does stem cell therapy work in dementia? There are two general approaches. The first involves the transplantation of undifferentiated (immature) cells whose subsequent development would be controlled by cues derived from the patient's brain. The use of a second approach is

more likely; in this method stem cells are grown, in a culture dish, into the desired type of neuron according to the disease being treated – thus the cells grown for Parkinson's disease would be different from those grown for Alzheimer's disease. These cells would be transplanted back into the brain of the person being treated as a neuronal graft. This approach requires a greater understanding than we yet have of how to culture cells into the desired cell type.[45]

To date, most work in this field has involved the treatment of Parkinson's disease and overall the results have been moderately encouraging, with no major risks emerging. There are still many unknowns to be resolved including long-term cell survival, risks of immunological rejection and, not least, logistical issues about supply of tissue and ethical concerns. It is likely to be at least 10 to 15 years before we know if stem cell therapy will be viable in the treatment of Alzheimer's disease. If it does work, it will probably be used in combination with drug treatments in a similar fashion to gene therapy.

Other treatments

There are many other treatments that are currently in varying stages of investigation and often feature in media reports. Some may have great potential, others will probably only have a limited effect or may never demonstrate sufficient benefit or safety for clinical use. These are listed in Table 13.1.

Table 13.1 Summary of selected treatments under investigation for Alzheimer's disease

Treatment	How it works	Potential effectiveness	Potential drawbacks	When available
1. Anti-amyloid agents				
Beta-amyloid vaccination (immunotherapy) e.g. bapineuzumab, solanezumab, gantenerumab, vanutide cridificar, CAD106	Increases the breakdown of beta-amyloid protein	Very effective; may halt the damage and result in improvement	Active vaccination more side effects than passive; side effects include malaise, pneumonia, angina, syncope, encephalitis	5–10 years if effective: bapineuzumab and solanezumab had negative Phase III trials; solanezumab and gantenerumab are part of DIAN study to prevent AD, vanutide cridificar Phase II trial due 2013
Gamma-secretase inhibitors e.g. semagacestat, tarenflurbil, avagacestat	Reduce the production of beta-amyloid protein	Very effective; may halt the damage and result in improvement	May need to be administered in pre-symptomatic state; selective gamma secretases need to be developed due to toxicity	10 years; Phase III trials either negative (tarenflurbil) or ceased due to toxicity (semagacestat)
Beta-secretase inhibitors e.g. LY288672, MK8931	Reduce the production of beta-amyloid protein	Very effective; may halt the damage and result in improvement	May need to be administered in prodromal AD; some agents impair cognition and function	5–10 years if effective; in Phase II trials

cont.

Treatment	How it works	Potential effectiveness	Potential drawbacks	When available
GSK inhibitors e.g. lithium, NP12	Reduce the production of amyloid and tau protein	Lithium may reduce risk of AD in bipolar patients; new drugs could be very effective	Lithium requires monitoring of blood levels and has tolerability concerns; new drugs are likely to have significant side effects	Lithium is available now but studies required will take 10–15 years, NP12 in Phase II studies
PBT2	Prevents the accumulation of amyloid by removing copper and zinc, which in turn inhibits amyloid-forming enzymes	Moderate – early studies show limited benefit; for combination therapy	Appears well tolerated in Phase II trials	5–10 years; in Phase II trials
CPHPC	Reduces serum amyloid protein blood levels, may reduce amyloid plaque formation	Very effective; may halt the damage and result in improvement	Appears to be well tolerated in Phase I trials but significant potential for adverse outcomes	10–20 years; in Phase I trials
Methylthioninium chloride TRx0014 (methylene blue)	Dissolves and inhibits formation of neurofibrillary tangles; inhibits tau aggregation	Moderate: early studies show greatest benefit in moderate AD	Hypertension, chest pain, dizziness, headache, discoloured urine	5–10 years; Phase II trials completed but unpublished

Treatment	How it works	Potential effectiveness	Potential drawbacks	When available
ELND005	Inhibition of beta-amyloid oligomer formation	Very effective; may halt the damage	Serious adverse effects including deaths resulted in cessation of higher doses of trial drug in late 2009	5–10 years; in Phase II trials on lower doses and for treatment of agitation and aggression
Receptor for Advanced Glycation End products (RAGE) e.g. PF-04494700, TTP-448	Binds to beta-amyloid protein and mediates its transport across the blood brain barrier	Very effective; may halt the damage	Well tolerated in Phase I/II trials	5–10 years; in Phase II trials, early results modest for PF-04494700
2. Neuroprotective agents				
Ampakines e.g. CX717, LY 451395	Increases the activity of nerve receptors in the brain that compensate for decreased production of glutamate	Moderate in theory but awaiting data; possibly useful in combination with CHEIs	No major side effects reported but research in doses higher than used in AD blocked by the FDA due to concerns on brain changes	5–10 years; currently in Phase II trials
Proline-rich polypeptide complex/ Colostrinin	An antioxidant; may prevent the formation of or dissolve amyloid plaques	Moderate; early studies show limited benefit	Sleeplessness but generally well tolerated	10 years, peptide components under investigation, requires Phase II studies

cont.

3. Neurorestorative approaches

Treatment	How it works	Potential effectiveness	Potential drawbacks	When available
Gene therapy e.g. CERE-110	Genetically modified cells implanted in the brain to stimulate nerve growth	Very effective; will replace damaged and dead cells; used with drugs that halt disease process	Unknown at present but could include brain haemorrhage, tumour formation, chronic pain	15–20 years; currently in Phase II trials
Stem cell neuronal grafts	Stem cells cultured to form specific neuronal cells deficient in AD are implanted in the brain as a neuronal graft	Very effective; will replace damaged and dead cells; used with drugs that halt disease process	Unknown at present but could include brain haemorrhage, tumour formation	20+ years

4. Neurotransmitters/receptors

Nicotinic acetylcholine receptor alpha 7 agonist (CHRNA7) e.g. ABT-126, EVP-6124	Increase nicotinic cholinergic pathways shown to improve cognition, may reduce inflammation	Modest effect non-specific to AD or dementia; used in combination with other drugs	Nausea, light-headedness, headache, sleep problems, dizziness	5–10 years; currently in Phase II trials

Treatment	How it works	Potential effectiveness	Potential drawbacks	When available
Monoamineoxidase-B (MAO-B) Inhibitors e.g. RO4602522, selegeline	MAO-B activity increases the production of toxic reactive free radicals that contribute to the pathogenesis of AD	Modest effect, used in combination with other drugs	Insomnia, hallucinations, orthostatic hypotension	RO4602522 Phase II studies occurring in patients with moderate AD and taking donepezil or rivastigmine; Phase III trials of selegeline show no benefit in AD
Serotonin 6 Receptor Antagonists e.g. AVN 101, SB742457, LU AE 58054	Enhances neurotransmission	Moderate; use in drug combinations	No reported serious adverse effects	5–10 years; in Phase II trials
5HT6 Agonist PRX-07034, SB-742457	Improves cognition by increasing levels of acetylcholine	Moderate; use in drug combinations	No reported serious adverse effects	5–10 years SB-742457 Phase II trials completed, awaiting results
Latrepirdine (Dimebon)	Used in Russia for 20 years; combined cholinesterase inhibitor and NMDA inhibitor	Moderate; early studies showed benefit similar to other cholinesterase inhibitors	Appears well tolerated	Phase III trials had mixed results leading to discontinuation of drug development in 2012

cont.

Treatment	How it works	Potential effectiveness	Potential drawbacks	When available
Histamine-3 receptor antagonist e.g. GSK 239512, ABT-288	Increases dopamine, acetylcholine and noradrenaline levels	Moderate, may improve cognition and alertness	Insomnia, diarrhoea, headache, muscle spasms, stomach discomfort	5–10 years; in Phase II trials
5. Other treatments				
Intranasal insulin	Enhances insulin signalling – memory loss in AD may be associated with low brain insulin	Moderate; early studies show benefit; will probably be used in combination with other treatments	Appears to be well tolerated	5–10 years; in Phase II trials
COGNIShunt	A pump implanted in the brain removes CSF to prevent toxic proteins from accumulating and forming plaques and tangles	Moderate – early studies show limited benefit; not likely to work by itself.	Infections of the pump and brain, headaches; invasive surgery for moderate benefit	5–10 years; Phase III trials completed, results not published, unlikely to be useful

Source: Taken from references 46–52.

Assistive technology

A range of assistive technologies to compensate for cognitive impairments due to dementia have emerged over the last few decades, particularly in recent years with advances in information technology. There are many innovative ideas but relatively few have been adequately evaluated yet. The list here is far from exhaustive and is intended to provide an indication of the direction research is heading.[53]

Prospective memory aids

Prospective memory aids are not just simple reminder systems; they are context-aware and use artificial intelligence to determine whether and when a reminder or guidance is necessary to assist the person with dementia. These aids are still in the early stages of development and although there are several commercially available products, they have not been adequately trialled in persons with dementia. 'Memory Glasses' is an example of a prospective memory aid in which a context-aware memory aid is embedded in a pair of spectacles. It has yet to be evaluated in clinical trials. The memory aid uses a variety of computer perception techniques to deliver a prompt to the user. The prompt has to be delivered at an appropriate time in order to avoid distracting the user during a task (such as when crossing a street) and when the user actually needs to know.

Retrospective memory aids

These memory aids allow the user to retrieve a record of what has happened in order to allow them to reconstruct memories. SenseCam, developed by Microsoft, is a wearable digital camera with a wide-angle lens designed to take photos passively while it is being worn. The user can bolster their autobiographical memory of events by viewing the photo images later. The SenseCam has had some limited evaluation in persons with dementia with some evidence that it can improve episodic memory. Researchers using SenseCam have suggested that memory technologies need to go beyond simply assisting accurate recall of events by fostering the involvement of support groups such as family members to strengthen interpersonal relationships.[54]

Language impairment aids

These aids are designed to compensate for the aphasic person's inability to follow written and verbal instructions. The 'Cook's Collage' is a video-based reminder system that displays the previous six steps completed in a

cooking task to reorient the user to the remainder of the activity. A small clinical trial showed promise and further trials are planned.[55]

Navigational aids

People with mild to moderate cognitive impairment are liable to get easily disoriented. A mobile phone-embedded device, 'Opportunity Knocks', uses a global position sensor (GPS) chip and Bluetooth, which learns the user's standard routes in the community. It alerts the person about navigational errors by making a knocking sound and it then works out the proper route. An Android application, iWander, using GPS and communication functions available via the smart phone, provides tracking of the location of the person with dementia and allow caregivers to provide assistance when needed. The system was shown to improve functional independence among people with dementia while decreasing the stress put on caregivers.[56]

Physiological sensors

Sensors can be used to monitor the person with dementia's vital signs, metabolism and to detect falls. Their main use is for person with dementia at home alone. Sensors can be attached to clothing and embedded in fabrics. The simplest type of sensor merely records information about the person with dementia, for example temperature and pulse, that is later played back. This is of limited utility. Newer devices have the capacity to monitor continuously in real time and transmit digital reports on a wide range of physiological parameters to family and professional caregivers with the intent of alerting them to changes from baseline measures of vital signs and metabolic function. This would then facilitate early intervention. Garments with embedded biosensors, so-called 'smart garments', have yet to be fully evaluated in persons with dementia but it is likely that some reconfiguration will be required to improve comfort and compliance.[57]

Advanced integrated sensor systems

These sensor systems fuse information from a network of sensors and apply artificial intelligence resulting in a more sophisticated level of supervision, guidance and feedback. CareWatch is a security system designed to alert caregivers about the person with dementia exiting the home. It consists of a security system control panel, a wireless receiver, and motion, door opening and bed occupancy sensors to alert the caregiver of both emergency and non-urgent situations through customisable text

or voice alarms. Early evaluation of the system has been positive without any major failures.

Integrating assistive technology into a functioning community environment has challenges. The Assistive Technology for Independence (AT4I) scheme introduced tailored packages of assistive technology into a sheltered housing development with 40 self-contained dwellings in Yorkshire, England. After user consultation, packages were developed and participants could choose one or more packages to suit their individual needs. The 'lifestyle reassurance package' consisted of bed and chair occupancy sensors, passive infra-red movement detectors, and door and electrical usage sensors. The 'security package' had a front door CCTV, intruder alarm, flood and extreme heat detectors. The 'falls package' had falls detectors and automatic light switches. An internet cafe was set up and proved to be very popular. The evaluation of the project was largely positive though it noted that in the initial stages of setting up the scheme there were teething difficulties with the technology as well as with the service providers understanding how to use the system.[58]

There are many challenges that need to be met before assistive technologies take up a mainstream role in dementia management. At present, most devices were originally designed for fit, younger people with static brain injuries; thus some of the specific issues confronting an older person with progressive cognitive impairment and other health problems have yet to be adequately met.

How will effective prevention and treatment of dementia affect our society?

The demographic imperative of an ageing society that has driven much of the research into various aspects of dementia care from a molecular to a societal level was discussed in Chapter 1. According to the 2009 World Alzheimer Report, the number of dementia cases in the world is predicted to increase from around 35.6 million in 2010 to 65.7 million in 2030 and to 115.4 million in 2050.[59] But what will it mean for society if by 2050 effective dementia therapies can both prevent the onset of dementia, halt the progression of early dementia, and possibly reverse some, if not all, of the damage done to come close to a 'cure'? If dementia is largely removed as the main cause of disability in older people, will they live longer in good health or will other serious conditions – cancer, arthritis, heart disease, diabetes, lung disease – simply become more apparent as causes of

death and disability? As dementia is now the main reason for admission to residential care, will there still be the same level of need for these facilities or could we look after even more people in their own homes?

These are all important questions that are not really answerable at present. Some authorities theorise that the natural lifespan for humans may be around 125 years.[60] Ideally, effective treatments for any illness will allow a person to live their natural lifespan with minimal disability and a good quality of life. But the availability of effective treatments would not necessarily mean that most people for whom they were suitable would use them. This might happen due to the cost (none of the new dementia drugs is likely to be cheap), the ignorance of doctors, patients and caregivers about the availability of treatment, a failure to detect dementia until a late stage (when treatments might have only limited benefit), or the refusal of some people to be treated. Some of this might be reduced with education about dementia, but I suspect that there will always be a significant number of untreated people. Even if only one third of the potential number of people with dementia in 2050 were to go untreated (and I believe that proportion is optimistic), this would still leave us with around 38 million untreated people, more than the number of people in the world with dementia in 2010!

If these problems were to be overcome and most people with dementia were to receive effective treatment, the inbuilt assumption is that they will die of other serious conditions. As implied in Chapter 1, there is a flaw in that argument. This is the tendency to ignore the rapid progress occurring in the prevention and treatment of most major medical conditions. In other words, older people are likely to potentially reduce their risks of succumbing to a whole range of potentially terminal illnesses. But effective treatments for other serious disabling, but not terminal conditions in old age – such as blindness from macular degeneration, nerve deafness, immobility from osteoarthritis and other causes of frailty – may not be discovered during the same time frame as treatment for dementia. This could result in an increasing population of alert but frail, possibly demoralised older people with disabilities who feel trapped by their incapacities.

Another possibility is that the new dementia treatments may not work indefinitely and may simply end up delaying the dementia for five to ten years. Does this mean that older people will die of other conditions before the dementia takes effect – a bit like it used to be 50 years ago? This may not be the case. We may delay the dementia, allowing people

to live a longer, healthier life until the dementia symptoms start to occur at an older age.

Summary

There are many exciting developments ahead in the prevention and treatment of dementia in general and Alzheimer's disease in particular. While this augers well, it is unlikely that any cures will become available for at least 20 years, if at all, and likely that many of those being treated will remain disabled with significant impairments. Despite the improvements, the number of older people with dementia will still increase over the next 20 or 30 years at least. Family caregivers will remain their primary source of support, even though the number of family caregivers potentially available to older people will diminish in the same time period due to declining fertility and marital rates.[61] Thus for the foreseeable future, systems to support persons with dementia and their caregivers will remain the cornerstone of dementia care.

APPENDIX 1

Telephone Helplines

Most of these phone numbers are only available from within the country under which they are listed.

Canada

Alzheimer Society of Canada
Toll free: 1800 616 8816

Canadian Dementia Action Network
1 604 822 7377

Veterans Affairs Canada
Toll free crisis helpline: 1800 268 7708

Ireland

Alzheimer Society of Ireland National Helpline
1800 341 341

Northern Ireland

Alzheimer's Society Northern Ireland Helpline
028 9066 4100 (9am to 5pm)

Scotland

Alzheimer Scotland Dementia Helpline
24 hour freephone: 0808 808 3000

Scottish Dementia Working Group
For people with dementia: 0141 418 3939

UK

Age UK Advice
0800 169 6565

Alzheimer's Society Helpline (England, Wales and Northern Ireland)
0300 222 11 22

Dementia UK Helpline
0845 257 9406 (Tuesdays and Thursdays, 11am
to 8.45pm, Saturdays 10am to 1pm)
Staffed by specialist mental health nurses.

NHS Carers Direct
Free confidential information and advice for carers for UK landlines or mobiles:
0808 802 0202 (9am to 8pm Monday to Friday, 11am to 4pm weekends)

US
Alzheimer's Association
24/7 Helpline: 1800 272 3900

Alzheimer's Disease Education and Referral (ADEAR) Center
Toll free: 1800 438 4380 (8.30am to 5pm Eastern
Standard Time, Monday to Friday)

National Council on Aging (Eldercare Locator)
1800 677 1116 (9am to 8pm Eastern Standard Time, Monday to Friday)

National Hotline for Veterans' Affairs benefits
1800 827 1000

Respite Care Locator Service
1919 490 5577

Veterans' Affairs Caregiver Support Line
1855 260 3274

Websites with Information About Accessing Services in Canada, Ireland, Scotland, the UK and the US

Canada

Alzheimer Society of Canada

www.alzheimer.ca/

The Alzheimer Society of Canada offers resources for people with dementia, caregivers, family members and health care practitioners in every province of Canada. It also provides a portal to First Link® which is a service that facilitates one-on-one or group support, referral to local health care providers and community services, meetings with other people in similar circumstances to exchange experiences, and help to plan your future. A second service available on the website is the Safely Home® Registry which assists police in finding a person who is lost and returning them safely to their home. It is a nationwide programme developed by the Alzheimer Society of Canada in partnership with the Royal Canadian Mounted Police.

Canadian Association of Retired Persons (CARP)

www.carp.ca

A Canadian website geared to life as a senior in Canada, CARP takes an online magazine approach to providing helpful information on topics relevant to retired Canadians. A source of helpful products and resources, this website also features advocacy, benefits, and community information for members.

Canadian Caregiver Coalition

www.ccc-ccan.ca

The national voice for the needs and interests of family caregivers, this is a bilingual, not-for-profit organisation made up of caregivers, caregiver support groups, national stakeholder organisations and researchers. Its work involves advocacy, research, education, resource development and communication.

Canadian Dementia Action Network (CDAN)
www.cdan.ca/
CDAN brings together Canada's world-class biomedical researchers and clinicians for the purpose of quickly identifying promising treatments for dementia.

Canadian Dementia Knowledge Translation Network
http://geriatricresearch.medicine.dal.ca/cdktn.htm
This is a network for translation and exchange of research in Alzheimer's disease and dementia.

Canadian Dementia Resource and Knowledge Exchange
www.dementiaknowledgebroker.ca/
The Canadian Dementia Resource and Knowledge Exchange is a network of people dedicated to improving the quality of life for persons with dementia and their family. It focuses on the national sharing of dementia resources and knowledge to support relationships among industry, researchers, clinicians, policy makers, persons with dementia, and care partners. You can pose questions on the website about all issues related to dementia care.

Canadian Senior Years
www.senioryears.com/index.html
This site was designed for Canadians over 50, providing information, articles, news and Canadian site links.

Seniors' Info
www.seniorsinfo.ca/en/welcome
This website, which is still under development, is part of a national project, the Collaborative Seniors' Portal Network, and has been developed through and by all three orders of government, and numerous seniors groups and service providers. to provide easy access for seniors, their families and service providers to important information.

Veterans Affairs Canada
www.veterans.gc.ca/eng
The website for Canadian veterans includes information about services and dementia.

Ireland
The Alzheimer Society of Ireland
www.alzheimer.ie/Home.aspx
The Alzheimer Society of Ireland website has information about dementia and about services for people with dementia and their caregivers.

Dementia Services Information and Development Centre

www.dementia.ie/

This is an Irish National Centre for excellence in dementia based at St James Hospital in Dublin. It provides services on education and training, information and consultancy, and research.

Trinity College Dublin, School of Social Work and Social Policy – Living with Dementia

www.socialwork-socialpolicy.tcd.ie/livingwithdementia/

Information about living with dementia pertinent to Ireland.

Northern Ireland

Alzheimer's Society Northern Ireland

www.alzheimers.org.uk/site/scripts/documents.php?categoryID=200140

The website of the Northern Ireland branch of the Alzheimer's Society, with information for regions of Northern Ireland.

Scotland

Alzheimer Scotland

www.alzscot.org/

Alzheimer Scotland helps people with dementia, their carers and families. This website has an abundance of information about dementia, how to obtain services, support for caregivers and long-term care.

NHS Health Scotland – Mental Health and Wellbeing in Late Life

www.healthscotland.com/topics/stages/healthy-ageing/mental-health-later-life.aspx

This is the web page of the NHS in Scotland that covers links to information about dementia and other mental health issues in late life.

The Scottish Dementia Working Group

www.sdwg.org.uk/

This is a campaigning group run by people with dementia in Alzheimer Scotland to improve services for people with dementia and to improve attitudes towards people with dementia. Membership is open to people with dementia.

Scottish Government – Dementia Information

www.scotland.gov.uk/Topics/Health/Services/Mental-Health/Dementia

This web page provides information about the 2010 Scotland Dementia Strategy and progress reports on its implementation and the 2011 Standards of Care action plan coordinated for the Scottish government by the Mental Welfare Commission for Scotland.

Well Scotland – Dementia Information
www.wellscotland.info/guidance/tamfs/later/dvdscript.aspx
This is the dementia section of the Scottish national mental health improvement website.

UK

Age UK
www.ageuk.org.uk/
Age UK is a charity formed from the amalgamation of Age Concern and Help The Aged. The Age UK Group provides services and support for older people in the UK. The website provides information about community and residential care for older people in the UK as well as information about assistive technology, insurance, finances, lifestyle issues and training opportunities.

Alzheimer's Society
www.alzheimers.org.uk/
This is the UK Alzheimer's Society website. It has a very good range of help sheets about various aspects of dementia that can be downloaded.

AT Dementia – information on assistive
technology for people with dementia
www.atdementia.org.uk/default.asp
This website brings together information about assistive technology that has the potential to support the independence and leisure opportunities of people with dementia.

Dementia UK
www.dementiauk.org/
This is a national charity committed to improving the lives of all people affected by dementia.

NHS Care at Home
www.nhs.uk/CarersDirect/guide/practicalsupport/Pages/Careathome.aspx
Government information about the type of support that is available including a search engine to find the closest services to where you live.

Paying for Care
www.payingforcare.org/
This is a website launched in 2011 designed to help individuals make more informed decisions about the arrangements and funding for their long-term care. The site is equally useful for powers of attorney and family members and friends. The site endeavours to give balanced, up-to-date advice on the complex subject of long-term care, specifically care payment, through careful, continuous research and collaboration with care fees experts and respected support organisations. It has information about regional care home fees, types

of local authority support, care entitlements and how to claim them, types of care, the care needs assessment, choosing a care home and care payment options. You can also chat with an advisor online.

US

AARP Internet Resources on Ageing
www.aarp.org/internetresources/
This is a one-stop shop for internet resources on ageing.

Alzheimer's Association
www.alz.org/
This is the website of the US Alzheimer's Association. On this site, you'll find information about the disease as well as about the Association's efforts in the US. An interesting page on the site contains balanced information about alternative therapies.

Alzheimer's Disease Education and Referral (ADEAR) Center
www.nia.nih.gov/alzheimers
This is a service of the US National Institute on Aging (NIA), which is one of the National Institutes of Health in the US. The purpose of the website is to provide information about Alzheimer's disease and related disorders. It publicises recent research findings and has an email service to notify all registrants of new information. Multimedia educational material is available for lay people, clinicians and academics. You can even pose questions to NIA experts and receive a personal email reply. Other information available includes a large recently revised bibliography, a list of current research trials in dementia and links to other worthwhile sites. While this site has an American focus, the quality of the general information about dementia is outstanding.

The ARCH National Respite Network
http://chtop.org/ARCH.html
The ARCH National Respite Network and Resource Center assists and promotes the development of quality respite and crisis care programmes; to help families locate respite and crisis care services in their communities; and to serve as a strong voice for respite in all forums.

Benefitscheckup
www.benefitscheckup.org/cf/index.cfm?partner_id=58
BenefitsCheckUp helps you find and enrol in public and private benefits programmes. You can also find an online application for Medicare's Extra Help. It's simple and free and always includes the most up-to-date information.

Caring Connections
www.caringinfo.org/i4a/pages/index.cfm?pageid=3284
Has downloads of state-specific forms for advance directives.

Center for Medicare and Medicaid Services

www.cms.gov

The agency oversees the Medicare and Medicaid programs.

Disability.gov

www.disability.gov

Disability.gov is a comprehensive federal website of disability-related government resources.

Eldercare Locator website

http://eldercare.gov/Eldercare.NET/Public/Index.aspx

The Eldercare Locator is a public service of the US Administration on Aging. It is designed to help older adults and their families and caregivers find their way through the maze of services for seniors by identifying trustworthy local support resources. The goal is to provide users with the information and resources that will help older persons live independently and safely in their homes and communities for as long as possible. It includes fact sheets on topics such as day care, assisted living, assistive technology, home health care and home modifications.

GovBenefits.gov

www.GovBenefits.gov

This is the official US government benefits website. It is a free, confidential tool that helps individuals find government benefits they may be eligible to receive.

The Huntington's Disease Society of America

www.hdsa.org/

Information on the genetic disorder, Huntington's disease.

National Clearinghouse for Long-term Care Information

www.longtermcare.gov/LTC/Main_Site/index.aspx

This website includes a state-by-state resource for finding community services.

National Council on Aging

www.ncoa.org/

The National Council on Aging is a non-profit service and advocacy organisation and a national voice for older Americans and the community organisations that serve them. It brings together non-profit organisations, businesses, and government to develop creative solutions that improve the lives of all older adults.

Social Security Administration

www.ssa.gov

The official site for Social Security. The website contains a wealth of information and resources including online databases and publications.

US Administration on Aging Alzheimer's Resource Room

www.agingcare.com/Support-Organizations/113676/The-Administration-on-Aging-Alzheimer-s-Resource-Room.htm

The US Administration on Aging's resource 'room' website provides families, carers and professionals with information about Alzheimer's disease, caregiving, working with and providing services to persons with Alzheimer's.

USA.gov for Seniors

www.usa.gov/Topics/Seniors.shtml

USA.gov for Seniors site helps users access all government sites that provide services for senior citizens.

Sites with scientific and medical information about dementia

Australian Institute of Health and Welfare

www.aihw.gov.au/

This is Australia's national agency for health and welfare statistics and information. It contains many reports on ageing, including the excellent 'Older Australians at a Glance'. There is also much statistical information about residential and community aged care, dementia and carers.

CogState

www.cogstate.com/

This is a computerised test of cognitive function available over the internet that can be accessed by the general public for a fee. The test is repeated over time and is alleged to be sensitive to early cognitive decline, though it cannot distinguish the cause. There is plenty of research being undertaken with CogState but at present it has yet to be validated for detecting dementia.

Cognitive Stimulation Therapy for Dementia

www.cstdementia.com/index.php

This website is by the team that developed cognitive stimulation therapy and provides good information about it.

DementiaGuide

www.dementiaguide.com/

A practical website about dementia to help people with Alzheimer's disease and their caregivers understand, recognise, record and track their symptoms through an interactive, online tool which is accessible with a subscription.

Dementia Collaborative Research Centres

www.dementia.unsw.edu.au/

The Dementia Collaborative Research Centres are an Australian Government initiative. They each focus on a different area of research.

Frontier – Frontotemporal Research Group
www.ftdrg.org
This is the website for the frontotemporal research group based at Prince of Wales Medical Research Institute in Sydney and it has excellent information about FTD for carers, patients and clinicians.

RUDAS Administration and Scoring Guide
http://www.health.qld.gov.au/tpch/html/rudas.asp
Information about how to administer and score the RUDAS.

MEDLINEplus – Alzheimer's Disease
www.nlm.nih.gov/medlineplus/alzheimersdisease.html
This site from the US National Library of Medicine has links to the most recent research findings about Alzheimer's disease as well as to other important American sites that contain information for consumers and health professionals.

The Merck Manual of Geriatrics
www.merck.com/pubs/mm_geriatrics/home.html
If you want to get some quick information about medical problems in old age, this is a good place to start.

National Institute on Aging
www.nia.nih.gov
NIA leads a broad scientific effort to understand the nature of ageing and to extend the healthy, active years of life.

National Institute of Neurological Disorders and Stroke – Alzheimer's Disease Information Page
www.ninds.nih.gov/disorders/alzheimersdisease/alzheimersdisease.htm
Another major American health institute that has an excellent site with mainly medical information about Alzheimer's disease. On another page, a very informative description of the life and death of neurons is provided that can be downloaded in full colour.

GPCOG Dementia Test
http://php.med.unsw.edu.au/gpcog/
An online version of this cognitive screening test along with information about dementia management.

The Nun Study
www.healthstudies.umn.edu/nunstudy/faq.jsp
Information about the Nun Study that has demonstrated that there are factors from early life which contribute to dementia.

International organisations relevant to dementia

Alzheimer's Disease International
www.alz.co.uk/
Alzheimer's Disease International is the umbrella organisation of Alzheimer associations around the world, which offer support and information to people with dementia and their carers. The website provides information about Alzheimer's disease, the global impact of Alzheimer's disease, research findings from the 10/66 Dementia Research Group, and how to find help. It also has a Cross Cultural Dementia Network that collates details of organisations that work with ethnic communities, rural populations, refugees and people of different sexual orientation.

A Dementia Voice
www.adementiavoice.com/
This is a website dedicated to people living with dementia to give them a place to express themselves online.

International Association of Gerontology and Geriatrics
www.iagg.com.br/webforms/index.aspx
This is the peak international body for age-related issues in health care and public policy.

International Psychogeriatric Association
www.ipa-online.org/
This is the peak international organisation for health professionals who treat older people with mental health problems.

APPENDIX 3

Books for Carers

The 36-Hour Day: A Family Guide to Caring for Persons with Alzheimer's Disease, Related Dementing Illnesses, and Memory Loss in Later Life (4th Edition) by Nancy Mace and Peter Rabins. Johns Hopkins University Press, Baltimore, 2006.

Alzheimer's and Other Dementias: Answers at your Fingertips (2nd Edition) by Harry Cayton, Nori Graham and James Warner. Class Publishing, London, 2008.

When your Loved One has Dementia: A Simple Guide for Caregivers by Joy A. Glenner, Jean M. Stehman, Judith Davagnino, Margaret J. Galante. Johns Hopkins University Press, Baltimore, 2005.

Alzheimer's Disease and Other Dementias: The Caregiver's Complete Survival Guide by Nataly Rubinstein. Two Harbors Press, Minneapolis, 2011.

Staying Afloat in a Sea of Forgetfulness: Common Sense Caregiving by Gary Joseph Leblanc. Xlibris Corporation, 2010.

Glossary

Acetylcholine: A neurotransmitter involved in learning and memory that is severely diminished in Alzheimer's disease.

Activities of daily living (ADL): Personal care activities necessary for everyday living, such as eating, bathing, grooming, dressing, and toileting.

Advance care directives (Living Wills): Written statements made by a competent person about what medical treatment they would like when they are no longer competent to make the decision.

Advocate: A person who acts on the behalf of another party.

Age-associated memory impairment: A decline in short-term memory that sometimes accompanies ageing.

Ageing in place: An approach that aims to provide residents with appropriate care and increased choice by allowing them to remain in the same aged care home regardless of their levels of care needs.

Agitation: Behaviour that is often accompanied by emotional distress and may include restlessness, vocal disruption and intrusiveness.

Alpha-synuclein: Protein found in Lewy bodies which occurs in dementia with Lewy bodies and Parkinson's disease.

Alzheimer's disease: The most common type of dementia amongst older people.

Amnestic disorders: A group of disorders characterised by loss of memory in the absence of other cortical dysfunction.

Amyloid plaque: Insoluble clumps of beta-amyloid protein found in the brains of people with Alzheimer's disease.

Amyloid precursor protein (APP): A large protein from which beta-amyloid is derived, found throughout the brain.

Antioxidants: Substances that remove free radicals which are thought to damage the brain.

Aphasia: Loss of language skills that can involve comprehension (receptive aphasia), ability to use language (expressive aphasia) or both.

Apolipoprotein E (APOE): A protein synthesised in the liver and brain that is involved in lipid metabolism and found to be associated with Alzheimer's disease.

Atrophy: Shrinkage, usually due to nerve cell death when it occurs in the brain.

Autonomy: A person's right to make decisions for themselves.

Behaviour management: Therapy targeted at specific behaviours in an attempt to extinguish unwanted behaviour and encourage desired behaviour.

Behavioural and psychological symptoms of dementia (BPSD): Symptoms of dementia that include mood disorders, psychosis, wandering, disruptive vocalisation, aggression and agitation.

Beta-amyloid protein: The protein that accumulates in amyloid plaques in people with Alzheimer's disease.

BPSD (see behavioural and psychological symptoms of dementia).

Brahmi: A popular Indian herb used to treat a range of nervous complaints including memory loss.

Brain scan: An investigation that shows a picture of the brain (see computerised tomography scan and magnetic resonance imaging).

Carer or caregiver: A person who looks after or gives care to a disabled person.

Central nervous system (CNS): The brain and spinal cord.

Cerebral haemorrhage: Stroke due to bleeding into the brain.

Cerebral infarction: Stroke due to loss of blood supply to the brain.

Cerebrospinal fluid (CSF): Fluid circulating around the brain and spinal cord that contains nutrients and removes toxins.

Cholinesterase inhibitors: Medications used to treat Alzheimer's disease that increase the availability of acetylcholine in the brain by inhibiting its breakdown.

Cognition: The mental activities associated with thinking, learning and memory.

Competency: Ability of a person to make rational decisions concerning personal affairs or welfare.

Computerised tomography (CT) scan: A computerised X-ray that gives a 3-D view of the body.

Confusion: A mental state caused by dementia, delirium and other conditions that involves impairment in thinking, awareness and concentration and is often associated with behaviour change.

Creutzfeldt-Jakob disease (CJD): A rare infectious disease that causes dementia.

CT scan (see computerised tomography)

Decision-making capacity: To have the capacity to make a decision, the person must be capable of understanding the nature of the decision and the effects that the decision will have upon the person and others.

Delirium (acute confusional state): A transient, global disorder of cognition that develops over days to weeks, usually due to an acute medical problem or medication.

Delusion: An unshakeable false belief that is out of keeping with the person's cultural or religious background.

Dementia: An acquired decline in memory and thinking (cognition) due to brain disease that results in significant impairment of personal, social or occupational function.

Dementia with Lewy Bodies: A type of degenerative dementia characterised by fluctuating level of consciousness, parkinsonism and visual hallucinations.

Depression: A mental disorder involving a lowering of mood and other negative emotions, loss of interests, reduced activities, sleep, appetite and weight changes.

Disorientation: Impairment in the person's awareness of who they are (person), where they are (place) or of when it is (time).

Double-blind placebo-controlled study: A research study in which an active treatment is compared with an inactive treatment and neither the patient nor the therapist knows which treatment is being given.

Elder abuse: Physical, psychological or financial harm committed against an older person.

Enduring power of attorney: A legal document by which a mentally competent person authorises someone to make financial decisions and sign papers on their behalf that contains a statement that it will continue when their mental capacity is lost.

Executive function: Higher-order functions of the brain that include organisation, planning, decision making and judgement.

Free radicals: Small molecules that damage the brain in oxidative metabolism.

Frontotemporal dementia: A type of degenerative dementia that mainly affects the frontal and temporal lobes of the brain.

Gene: Genes are made up of four chemicals arranged in various patterns on the chromosome in the nucleus of each cell; they direct the manufacture of every enzyme, hormone and other protein in the body.

Geriatrician: A physician who specialises in treating older people.

Guardian: A legally appointed person who is a substitute decision-maker for a mentally incompetent person.

Hallucination: A perception without a stimulus.

Hippocampus: Part of the brain important in memory function.

Huntington's disease: A hereditary disorder that causes involuntary movements, personality change and dementia.

Impairment: Objective weakening, damage or deterioration as a result of injury or disease.

Incidence: The number of new cases of a disease in a defined population over a specific period of time.

Incontinence: Loss of control of bladder and/or bowel function.

Instrumental activities of daily living (IADL): Higher-order activities that include shopping, managing finances, cooking and housework.

Magnetic resonance imaging (MRI): A type of computerised scan that uses strong electromagnetic fields to provide a 3-D image.

Memory: The ability to remember past experiences.

Memory clinic: A clinic that specialises in the assessment and management of people with disorders of memory.

Mild cognitive impairment (MCI): Mild memory and other cognitive changes, more severe than normal ageing but not sufficient to be regarded as dementia.

Mini Mental State Examination (MMSE): A commonly used standardised test of cognitive function.

MRI scan (see magnetic resonance imaging).

Multidisciplinary team: A clinical team composed of members from different disciplines, such as medicine, nursing, occupational therapy, physical therapy and psychology.

Music therapy: A type of therapy that uses music to relieve symptoms of depression, agitation and distress.

Neurodegeneration: Progressive degeneration and death of nerve cells.

Neurofibrillary tangles: Composed of a protein called tau, and found in nerve cells in Alzheimer's disease and frontotemporal dementia.

Neuroimaging: Brain scans, for example, computerised tomography (CT), magnetic resonance imaging (MRI).

Neurologist: A physician who specialises in disorders of the nervous system.

Neuron: Nerve cell.

Neuropathology: The study of diseases of the nervous system, usually involving microscopic examination.

Neuropsychologist: A psychologist with training to perform and interpret standardised tests of cognition and mental functioning.

Neurotransmitter: A chemical messenger in the brain.

Normal pressure hydrocephalus: A type of dementia caused by blockage in the flow of cerebrospinal fluid (CSF) in the brain resulting in enlarged ventricles.

Old age psychiatrist (see psychogeriatrician).

Paranoia: Suspiciousness.

Parkinson's disease: A degenerative disease of the brain that results in slowing of movements, tremor, muscular rigidity and, usually, mental changes.

Parkinsonism: Slowing of movements, tremor and/or muscular rigidity.

PEG (percutaneous endoscopic gastrostomy) tube: A tube placed through the abdominal wall into the stomach to allow tube feeding.

Perseveration: The constant repetition of a meaningless word or phrase.

Person-centred care: An approach to care that views the person with dementia as a unique individual who has feelings, had a life before the illness, and whose wellbeing will be influenced by their psychosocial environment.

Pharmacotherapy: Drug therapy, medication.

Pick's disease: A type of frontotemporal dementia.

Placebo: An inactive treatment ('sugar pill') used for comparison with a new treatment to see if it works.

Placement: Transfer of an elderly person to a residential facility such as a nursing home, residential hospital or supervised hostel.

Plaques (see amyloid plaque).

Polypharmacy: Prescription of multiple drugs in the same patient with the potential for drug–drug interactions and adverse effects.

Power of attorney (POA): A legal document by which a mentally competent person authorises someone to make financial decisions and sign legal papers on their behalf. In some jurisdictions this might include personal care decisions.

Prevalence: The number of cases of a disease existing in a given population.

Prions: Small glycoproteins with infectious qualities found in Creutzfeldt-Jakob disease.

Progressive supranuclear palsy (PSP): Rare subcortical dementia involving gaze abnormalities, parkinsonism and unsteady walking.

Psychogeriatrician: A psychiatrist who specialises in treating older people with mental disorders.

Psychosis: A mental condition characterised by delusions and/or hallucinations in which the person has lost touch with reality.

Psychotropic drugs: Drugs that are used to treat the psychological and behavioural aspects of dementia.

Reality orientation: A type of therapy used in moderate–severe dementia to improve memory and orientation.

Receptor: A docking site on a nerve cell where neurotransmitters work.

Reminiscence therapy: A therapy used in dementia to invoke pleasant life memories, provide distraction and mental stimulation.

Respite care: Temporary formal care of a person with dementia to give the carer a rest.

Risk factors: Factors associated with a disease process.

Senile dementia: An outdated term once used to refer to any form of dementia that occurred in older people.

Senility: An outdated term that implies that mental deterioration and dementia is a part of normal ageing.

Statins: Medication that is used to reduce cholesterol levels that may help in preventing Alzheimer's disease.

Subcortical dementia: Dementia commencing in or mainly affecting areas of the brain below the cortex, for example, Huntington's disease, Parkinson's disease.

Substitute decision-maker: The person who makes decisions on behalf of a mentally incompetent person.

Sundowning: Agitated behaviour that characteristically occurs in late afternoon and early evening.

Support group: A group that provides emotional support to carers.

Synapse: The gap between nerve cells where neurotransmitters convey messages between nerves.

Tangles (see neurofibrillary tangles).

Tau protein: The protein found in neurofibrillary tangles.

Testamentary capacity: Capacity to make a will.

Tube feeding: Use of a feeding tube either through the nose or abdominal wall (see PEG tube) when a person is unable to swallow safely.

Validation therapy: A therapy that assists in communication with moderate–severe dementia by validating the person's emotions.

Vascular dementia: A type of dementia due to damage caused by blood vessel disease in the brain.

Wandering: A term that encompasses several types of behavioural changes found in dementia including restlessness, aimless walking and goal-directed walking.

Notes

Chapter 1

1. *CIA The World Fact Book*. Available at https://www.cia.gov/library/publications/the-world-factbook/geos/countrytemplate_xx.html, accessed on 22 December 2012.

2. *CIA The World Fact Book*. Available at https://www.cia.gov/library/publications/the-world-factbook/geos/countrytemplate_xx.html, accessed on 22 December 2012.

3. World Health Organization (1992) *The ICD-10 Classification of Mental and Behavioural Disorders: Diagnostic Criteria for Research*. Geneva: World Health Organization. Available at www.who.int/classifications/icd/en/GRNBOOK.pdf, accessed on 22 December 2012.

4. Winblad, B., Palmer, K., Kivipelto, M. *et al.* (2004) 'Mild Cognitive Impairment – beyond controversies, towards a consensus: report of the International Working Group on Mild Cognitive Impairment.' *Journal of Internal Medicine 256*, 240–246.

5. Park, D.C. and Reuter-Lorenz, P. (2009) 'The adaptive brain: aging and neurocognitive scaffolding.' *Annual Reviews in Psychology 60*, 173–196.

6. Park, D.C. and Reuter-Lorenz, P. (2009) 'The adaptive brain: aging and neurocognitive scaffolding.' *Annual Reviews in Psychology 60*, 173–196.

7. Alzheimer's Disease International (2009) *World Alzheimer Report 2009*. Edited by M. Prince and J. Jackson. Available at www.alz.co.uk/research/world-report, accessed on 8 December 2012.

8. Alzheimer's Disease International (2009) *World Alzheimer Report 2009*. Edited by M. Prince and J. Jackson. Available at www.alz.co.uk/research/world-report, accessed on 8 December 2012.

9. Access Economics (2009) 'Keeping dementia front of mind: incidence and prevalence 2009–2050.' Available at www.fightdementia.org.au/research-publications/access-economics-reports.aspx, accessed on 31 March 2013.

10. Matthews, F., Brayne, C., Medical Research Council Cognitive Function and Ageing Study Investigators (2005) 'The incidence of dementia in England and Wales: findings from the five identical Sites of the MRC CFA Study.' *PLoS Med 2*, 8, e193. doi:10.1371/journal.pmed.0020193.

11. Schrijvers, E.M., Verhaaren, B.F., Koudstaal, P.J., Hofman, A., Ikram, M.A. and Breteler, M.M. (2012) 'Is dementia incidence declining? Trends in dementia incidence since 1990 in the Rotterdam Study.' *Neurology 78*, 19, 1456–63.

12. Vickland, V., Morris, T., Draper, B., Low, L.F. and Brodaty, H. (2012) 'Modelling the impact of interventions to delay the onset of dementia in Australia. A report for Alzheimer's Australia.'

http://www.fightdementia.org.au/common/files/NAT/201212_NAT_AAnumbered Pub_Paper30final.pdf, accessed on 8 December 2012.

13. Shanks, M., Kivipelto, M., Bullock, R., Lane, R. (2009) Cholinesterase inhibition: is there evidence for disease-modifying effects? *Current Medical Research & Opinion 25*, 10, 2439–46.

14. Australian Institute of Health and Welfare (2012) *Dementia in Australia.* Canberra: AIHW.

15. Alzheimer's Disease International (2009) *World Alzheimer Report 2009.* Edited by M. Prince and J. Jackson. Available at www.alz.co.uk/research/world-report, accessed on 8 December 2012.

16. World Health Organization (2008) *The Global Burden of Disease: 2004 Update.* Available at www.who.int/healthinfo/global_burden_disease/GBD_report_2004update_full.pdf, accessed on 22 December 2012.

17. Alzheimer's Disease International (2010) *World Alzheimer Report 2010: The Global Economic Impact of Dementia.* Edited by A. Wimo and M. Prince. Available at www.alz.co.uk/research/world-report, accessed on 8 December 2012.

18. Alzheimer's Disease International (2010) *World Alzheimer Report 2010: The Global Economic Impact of Dementia.* Edited by A. Wimo and M. Prince. Available at www.alz.co.uk/research/world-report, accessed on 8 December 2012.

19. Alzheimer's Disease International (2010) *World Alzheimer Report 2010: The Global Economic Impact of Dementia.* Edited by A. Wimo and M. Prince. Available at www.alz.co.uk/research/world-report, accessed on 8 December 2012.

20. Access Economics (2009) 'Making choices: future dementia care: projections, problems and preferences. Report for Alzheimer's Australia.' Available at www.fightdementia.org.au/research-publications/access-economics-reports.aspx, accessed on 31 March 2013.

21. Luengo-Fernandez, R., Leal, J. and Gray, A. (2010) *Dementia 2010.* Oxford: The Health Economics Research Centre, University of Oxford.

22. Hurd, M.D., Martorell, P., Delavande. A. et al. (2013) 'Monetary costs of dementia in the United States.' *New England Journal of Medicine 368*, 14 April, 4.

23. Murray, C.J., Vos, T., Lozano, R. et al. (2012) 'Disability-adjusted life years (DALYs) for 291 diseases and injuries in 21 regions, 1990–2010: a systematic analysis for the Global Burden of Disease Study 2010.' *Lancet 380*, 9859, 2197–2223.

24. Department of Health (2009) Living Well with Dementia: A National Dementia Strategy. Available at www.dh.gov.uk/en/Publicationsandstatistics/Publications/PublicationsPolicyAndGuidance/DH_094058, accessed on 15 July 2012.

25. Alzheimer's Society (2009) 'Dementia research funding must triple, say experts.' 30 June. Available at www.alzheimers.org.uk/site/scripts/press_article.php?pressReleaseID=364, accessed on 24 March 2013.

26. Voice of America (2012) 'US launches campaign against Alzheimer's including prevention drug trials.' 15 May. Available at www.voanews.com/content/new_us_initiative_takes_aim_at_alzheimers_disease/666646.html, accessed on 7 March 2013.

Chapter 2

1. Daviglus, M.L., Bell, C.C., Berrettini, W. *et al.* (2010) 'National Institutes of Health State-of-the-Science Conference Statement: Preventing Alzheimer's Disease and Cognitive Decline.' 26–28 April. *NIH Consens State Sci Statements 27*, 4, 1–27.

2. Coley, N., Andrieu, S., Gardette, V. *et al.* (2008) 'Dementia prevention: methodological explanations for inconsistent results.' *Epidemiologic Reviews 30*, 35–66.

3. Australian Bureau of Statistics (1998) *Suicides 1921–1998.* Cat. no. 3309.0. Canberra: ABS. Available at www.ausstats.abs.gov.au/Ausstats/subscriber.nsf/0/B677BAE5E1AC

97E5CA2568BD0012ECBC/$File/33090_1921%20to%201998.pdf, accessed on 22 December 2012.

4. Schenk, D., Barbour, R., Dunn, W. *et al.* (1999) 'Immunization with amyloid-β attenuates Alzheimer-disease-like pathology in the PDAPP mouse.' *Nature 400*, 173–177.

5. Bayer, A.J., Bullock, R., Jones, R.W. *et al.* (2005) 'Evaluation of the safety and immunogenicity of synthetic Abeta42 (AN1792) in patients with AD.' *Neurology 64*, 94–101.

6. Vellas, B., Black, R., Thal, L.J. *et al.* (2009) 'Long-term follow-up of patients immunized with AN1792: reduced functional decline in antibody responders.' *Current Alzheimer Research 6*, 2, 144–151.

7. Winblad, B., Andreasen, N., Minthon, L. *et al.* (2012) 'Safety, tolerability, and antibody response of active A^2 immunotherapy with CAD106 in patients with Alzheimers disease: randomised, double-blind, placebo-controlled, first-in-human study.' *Lancet Neurology 11*, 7, 597–604. doi: 10.1016/S1474-4422(12)70140-0.

8. Vickland, V., McDonnell, G., Werner, J. *et al.* (2010) 'A computer model of dementia prevalence in Australia: foreseeing outcomes of delaying dementia onset, slowing disease progression, and eradicating dementia types.' *Dementia & Geriatric Cognitive Disorders 29*, 123–130.

9. Colantuoni, E., Surplus, G., Hackman, A. et al. (2010) 'Web-based application to project the burden of Alzheimer's disease.' *Alzheimer's & Dementia 6*, 425–428.

10. Barnes, D.E. and Yaffe, K. (2011) 'The projected effect of risk factor reduction on Alzheimer's disease prevalence.' *Lancet Neurology 10*, 819–828.

11. Borenstein, A.R., Copenhaver, C. and Mortimer, J.A. (2006) 'Early life risk factors for Alzheimer disease.' *Alzheimer Disease & Associated Disorders 20*, 63–72.

12. Ritchie, K., Jaussent, I., Stewart, R. *et al.* (2011) 'Adverse childhood environment and late-life cognitive functioning.' *International Journal of Geriatric Psychiatry 26*, 503–510.

13. Butterworth, P., Cherbuin, N., Sachdev, P., Anstey, K.J. (2012) 'The association between financial hardship and amygdala and hippocampal volumes: results from the PATH through life project.' *Social Cognitive and Affective Neuroscience 7*, 5, 548–556.

14. McGurn, B., Deary, I.J. and Starr, J.M. (2008) 'Childhood cognitive ability and risk of late-onset Alzheimer and vascular dementia.' *Neurology 71*, 1051–1056.

15. Norton, M.C., Østbye, T., Smith, K.R. *et al.* (2009) 'Early parental death and late-life dementia risk: findings from the Cache County Study.' *Age and Ageing 38*, 3, 340–343.

16. Alzheimer's Disease International (2009) World Alzheimer Report 2009. Edited by M. Prince and J. Jackson. Available at www.alz.co.uk/research/world-report, accessed on 8 December 2012.

17. Masaki, K.H., Losonczy, K.G., Izmirlian, G. *et al.* (2000) 'Association of Vitamin E and C supplement use with cognitive function and dementia in elderly men.' *Neurology 54*, 1265–1272.

18. Engelhart, M.J., Geerlings, M.I., Ruitenberg, A. *et al.* (2002) 'Dietary intake of antioxidants and risk of Alzheimer disease.' *JAMA 287*, 24, 3223–3229.

19. Morris, M.C., Evans, D.A., Bienias, J.L. *et al.* (2002) 'Vitamin E and cognitive decline in older persons.' *Archives of Neurology 59*, 7, 1125–1132.

20. Middleton, L.E. and Yaffe, K. (2009) 'Promising strategies for the prevention of dementia.' *Archives of Neurology 66*, 10, 1210–1215.

21. Devore, E.E., Grodstein, F., van Rooij, F.J. *et al.* (2010) 'Dietary antioxidants and long-term risk of dementia.' *Archives of Neurology 67*, 7, 819–825.

22. von Arnim, C.A.F., Herbolsheimer, F., Nikolaus, T. *et al.* (2012) 'Dietary antioxidants and dementia in a population-based case-control study among older people in south Germany.' *Journal of Alzheimer's Disease.* doi: 10.3233/JAD-2012-120634.

23. Kim, D.S., Kim, J.Y. and Han, Y. (2012) 'Curcuminoids in neurodegenerative diseases.' *Recent Patents on CNS Drug Discovery 7*, 3, 184–204.

24. Ringman, J.M., Frautschy, S.A., Teng, E. *et al.* (2012) 'Oral curcumin for Alzheimer's disease: tolerability and efficacy in a 24-week randomized, double blind, placebo-controlled study.' *Alzheimer's Research & Therapy 4*, 43. doi: 10.1186/alzrt146

25. Ridley, N.J., Draper, B. and Withall, A. (2013) 'Alcohol-related dementia: an update of the evidence.' *Alzheimer's Research & Therapy 5*, 3. Available at: http://alzres.com/content/5/1/3.

26. Withall, A. and Draper, B. (2009) 'What is the burden of younger onset dementia in Australia?' *International Psychogeriatrics 21*, Suppl. 2, S26.

27. Ruitenberg, A., van Swieten, J.C., Witteman, J.C.M. *et al.* (2002) 'Alcohol consumption and risk of dementia: the Rotterdam Study.' *Lancet 359*, 9303, 281–286.

28. Truelsen, T., Thudium, D. and Grønbæk, M. (2002) 'Amount and type of alcohol and risk of dementia: the Copenhagen city heart study.' *Neurology 59*, 1313–1319

29. Desideri, G., Kwik-Uribe, C., Grassi, D. *et al.* (2012) 'Benefits in cognitive function, blood pressure, and insulin resistance through cocoa flavanol consumption in elderly subjects with mild cognitive impairment: the Cocoa, Cognition, and Aging (CoCoA) Study.' *Hypertension 60*, 794–801.

30. Low, L.-F., Yap, M.H.W. and Brodaty, H. (2010) 'Will testing for apolipoprotein E assist in tailoring dementia risk reduction? A review.' *Neuroscience and Biobehavioral Reviews 34*, 408–437.

31. Hoang, T., Barnes, D., Byers, A., Yaffe, K. (2012) '20-Year alcohol consumption patterns and cognitive impairment in older women.' Alzheimer's Association International Conference, 14–19 July. Vancouver, Canada.

32. Lang, I., Langa, K., Wallace, R. and Llewellyn, D. (2012) 'Heavy episodic drinking and risk of cognitive decline in older adults.' Alzheimer's Association International Conference, 14–19 July. Vancouver, Canada.

33. Seshadri, S. (2006) 'Elevated plasma homocysteine levels: risk factor or risk marker for the development of dementia and Alzheimer's disease?' *Journal of Alzheimer's Disease 9*, 393–398.

34. Smith, A.D., Smith, S.M., de Jager, C.A. *et al.* (2010) Homocysteine-lowering by B Vitamins slows the rate of accelerated brain atrophy in mild cognitive impairment: a randomized controlled trial.' *PLoS ONE 5*, 9, e12244. doi:10.1371/journal.pone.0012244.

35. Whitrow, M.J., Moore, V.M., Rumbold, A.R. and Davies M.J. (2009) 'Effect of supplemental folic acid in pregnancy on childhood asthma: a prospective birth cohort study.' American *Journal of Epidemiology 170*, 1486–1493.

36. Sydenham, E., Dangour, A.D. and Lim, W.-S. (2012) 'Omega 3 fatty acid for the prevention of cognitive decline and dementia.' *Cochrane Database of Systematic Reviews*, Issue 6. Art. No.: CD005379. doi: 10.1002/14651858.CD005379.pub3.

37. Barberger-Gateau, P., Letenneur, L., Deschamps, V. *et al.* (2002) 'Fish, meat, and risk of dementia: cohort study.' *British Medical Journal 325*, 932–933.

38. Sydenham, E., Dangour, A.D., Lim, W.-S. (2012) 'Omega 3 fatty acid for the prevention of cognitive decline and dementia.' *Cochrane Database of Systematic Reviews*, Issue 6. Art. No.: CD005379. doi: 10.1002/14651858.CD005379.pub3.

39. Dixon, L.B., Cronin, F.J. and Krebs-Smith, S.M. (2001) 'Let the pyramid guide your food choices: capturing the total diet concept.' *Journal of Nutrition 131*, 461S–472S.

40. Willett, W.C. (1995) 'Mediterranean diet pyramid: a cultural model for healthy eating.' *American Journal of Clinical Nutrition 61*, 6, 1402S–6S.

41. Scarmeas, N., Luchsinger, J.A., Schupf, N. *et al.* (2009) 'Physical activity, diet, and risk of Alzheimer disease.' *JAMA 302*, 6, 627–637.

42. Feart, C., Samieri, C., Rondeau, V. *et al.* (2009) 'Adherence to a Mediterranean diet, cognitive decline, and risk of dementia.' *JAMA 302*, 6, 638–648.

43. Okereke, O.I., Rosner, B.A., Kim, D.H. *et al.* (2012) 'Dietary fat types and 4-year cognitive change in community-dwelling older women.' *Annals of Neurology 72*, 1, 124–34.

44. Gouveri, E.T., Tzavara, C., Drakopanagiotakis, F. *et al.* (2011) 'Mediterranean diet and metabolic syndrome in an urban population: the Athens Study.' *Nutrition in Clinical Practice 26*, 5, 598–606.

45. Tognon, G., Rothenberg, E., Eiben, G. *et al.* (2011) 'Does the Mediterranean diet predict longevity in the elderly? A Swedish perspective.' *Age 33*, 3, 439–450.

46. Etgen, T., Sander, D., Bickel, H. *et al.* (2012) 'Vitamin D deficiency, cognitive impairment and dementia: a systematic review and meta-analysis.' *Dementia & Geriatric Cognitive Disorders 33*, 5, 297–305.

47. Etgen, T., Sander, D., Bickel, H. *et al.* (2012) 'Vitamin D deficiency, cognitive impairment and dementia: a systematic review and meta-analysis.' *Dementia & Geriatric Cognitive Disorders 33*, 5, 297–305.

48. Cao, C., Cirrito, J.R., Lin, X. *et al.* (2009) 'Caffeine suppresses amyloid-beta levels in plasma and brain of Alzheimer's disease transgenic mice.' *Journal of Alzheimer's Disease 17*, 681–697.

49. Maia, L. and de Mendonca, A. (2002) 'Does caffeine intake protect from Alzheimer's disease?' *European Journal of Neurology 9*, 4, 377–82.

50. Valenzuela, M.J. (2008) 'Brain reserve and the prevention of dementia.' *Current Opinion in Psychiatry 21*, 296–302.

51. Barnes, D.E. and Yaffe, K. (2011) 'The projected effect of risk factor reduction on Alzheimer's disease prevalence.' *Lancet Neurology 10*, 819–828.

52. Snowdon, D. 'The Nun Study – frequently asked questions.' Available at www.healthstudies.umn.edu/nunstudy/faq.jsp, accessed on 11 January 2010.

53. Whalley, L.J., Starr, J.M., Athawes, R. *et al.* (2000) 'Childhood mental ability and dementia.' *Neurology 28*, 55, 10, 1455–9.

54. Schofield, P. (1999) 'Alzheimer's disease and brain reserve.' *Australasian Journal on Ageing 18*, 1, 10–14.

55. Helmes, E., Ostbye, T. and Steenhuis, R.E. (2011) 'Incremental contribution of reported previous head injury to the prediction of diagnosis and cognitive functioning in older adults.' *Brain Injury 25*, 4, 338–347.

56. Editorial (2009) 'Butting heads.' *Nature Neuroscience 12*, 1475.

57. Valenzuela, M.J. (2008) 'Brain reserve and the prevention of dementia.' *Current Opinion in Psychiatry 21*, 296–302.

58. Lin, F.R., Metter, E.J., O'Brien, R.J. *et al.* (2011) 'Hearing loss and incident dementia.' *Archives of Neurology 68*, 214–220.

59. Willis, S.L., Tennstedt, S.L., Marsiske, M., *et al.* (2006) 'Long-term effects of cognitive training on everyday functional outcomes in older adults.' *JAMA 296*, 2805–2814.

60. Wilson, R.S., Segawa, E., Boyle, P.A. and Bennett, D.A. (2012) 'Influence of late-life cognitive activity on cognitive health.' *Neurology 78*, 1123–1129.

61. Friedland, R.P., Fritsch, T., Smyth, K.A. *et al.* (2001) 'Patients with Alzheimer's disease have reduced activities in midlife compared with healthy control-group members.' *PNAS 98*, 3440–3445.

62. Lautenschlager, N.T., Cox, K.L., Flicker, L. *et al.* (2008) 'Effect of physical activity on cognitive function in older adults at risk for Alzheimer disease: a randomized trial.' *JAMA 300*, 1027–1037.

63. Barnes, D.E. and Yaffe, K. (2011) 'The projected effect of risk factor reduction on Alzheimer's disease prevalence.' *Lancet Neurology 10*, 819–828.

Chapter 3

1. Jonsson, T. *et al.* (2012) 'A mutation in APP protects against Alzheimer's disease and age-related cognitive decline.' *Nature 488*, 69–99 (2 August). doi: 10.1038/nature11283.

2. Liddell, M.B., Lovestone, S. and Owen, M.J. (2001) 'Genetic risk of Alzheimer's disease: advising relatives.' *British Journal of Psychiatry 178*, 7–11.

3. Liddell, M.B., Lovestone, S. and Owen, M.J. (2001) 'Genetic risk of Alzheimer's disease: advising relatives.' *British Journal of Psychiatry 178*, 7–11.

4. Liddell, M.B., Lovestone, S. and Owen, M.J. (2001) 'Genetic risk of Alzheimer's disease: advising relatives.' *British Journal of Psychiatry 178*, 7–11.

5. Low, L.-F., Yap, M.H.W. and Brodaty, H. (2010) 'Will testing for apolipoprotein E assist in tailoring dementia risk reduction? A review.' *Neuroscience and Biobehavioral Reviews 34*, 408–437.

6. National Institute on Aging/Alzheimer's Association Working Group (1996) 'Apolipoprotein E genotyping in Alzheimer's disease.' *Lancet 347*, 1091–1095.

7. Frontier – Frontotemporal Dementia Research Group (undated) 'What is frontotemporal dementia?' Available at www.ftdrg.org/caregivers/ftd/, accessed on 24 February 2010.

8. van Swieten, J.C., Rosso, S.M., Heutink, P. (2010) 'MAPT-related disorders.' *GeneReviews.* Available at www.ncbi.nlm.nih.gov/books/NBK1505/, accessed on 29 December 2012.

9. DeJesus-Hernandez, M., Mackenzie, I.R., Boeve, B.F. *et al.* (2011) 'Expanded GGGGCC Hexanucleotide repeat in noncoding region of C9ORF72 causes chromosome 9p-linked FTD and ALS.' *Neuron 72*, 2, 245–256.

10. Renton, A.E., Majounie, E., Waite, A. *et al.* (2011) 'A hexanucleotide repeat expansion in C9ORF72 is the cause of chromosome 9p21-linked ALS-FTD.' *Neuron 72*, 2, 257–268.

11. Lesnik Oberstein, S.A.J., Boon, E.M.J. and Terwindt, G.M. (2012) 'CADASIL.' GeneReviews. Available at www.ncbi.nlm.nih.gov/books/NBK1500/, accessed on 29 December 2012.

12. Schmidt, R., Schmidt, H. and Fazekas, F. (2000) 'Vascular risk factors in dementia.' *Journal of Neurology 247*, 81–87.

13. Middleton, L.E. and Yaffe, K. (2009) 'Promising strategies for the prevention of dementia.' *Archives of Neurology 66*, 10, 1210–1215.

14. Kivipelto, M., Helkala, E.L., Laakso, M.P. *et al.* (2001) 'Midlife vascular risk factors and Alzheimer's disease in later life: longitudinal, population based study.' *British Medical Journal 322*, 7300, 1447–1451.

15. Barnes, D.E. and Yaffe, K. (2011) 'The projected effect of risk factor reduction on Alzheimer's disease prevalence.' *Lancet Neurology 10*, 819–828.

16. Barnes, D.E. and Yaffe, K. (2011) 'The projected effect of risk factor reduction on Alzheimer's disease prevalence.' *Lancet Neurology 10*, 819–828.

17. Forette, F., Seux, M.L., Staessen, J.A., *et al.* (2002) 'The prevention of dementia with antihypertensive treatment: new evidence from the Systolic Hypertension in Europe (Syst-Eur) study.' *Archives of Internal Medicine 14*, 162, 18, 2046–2052.

18. PROGRESS Collaborative Group (2001) 'Randomised trial of a perindopril-based blood pressure lowering regimen among 6105 individuals with previous stroke or transient ischaemic attack.' *Lancet 358*, 9287,1033–1041.

19. Middleton, L.E. and Yaffe, K. (2009) 'Promising strategies for the prevention of dementia.' *Archives of Neurology 66*, 10, 1210–1215.

20. Barnes, D.E. and Yaffe, K. (2011) 'The projected effect of risk factor reduction on Alzheimer's disease prevalence.' *Lancet Neurology 10*, 819–828.

21. Kirshner, H.S. (2009) 'Vascular dementia: a review of recent evidence for prevention and treatment.' *Current Neurology and Neuroscience Reports 9*, 437–442.

22. Almeida, O.P., Hulse, G.K., Lawrence, D. *et al.* (2002) 'Smoking as a risk factor for Alzheimer's disease: contrasting evidence from a systematic review of case-control and cohort studies.' *Addiction 97*, 1, 15–28.
23. Barnes, D.E. and Yaffe, K. (2011) 'The projected effect of risk factor reduction on Alzheimer's disease prevalence.' *Lancet Neurology 10*, 819–828.
24. Barnes, D.E. and Yaffe, K. (2011) 'The projected effect of risk factor reduction on Alzheimer's disease prevalence.' *Lancet Neurology 10*, 819–828.
25. Stewart, R. and Liolitsa, D. (1999) 'Type 2 diabetes mellitus, cognitive impairment and dementia.' *Diabetic Medicine 12*, 2, 93–112.
26. Low, L.-F., Yap, M.H.W. and Brodaty, H. (2010) 'Will testing for apolipoprotein E assist in tailoring dementia risk reduction? A review.' *Neuroscience and Biobehavioral Reviews 34*, 408–437.
27. Barnes, D.E. and Yaffe, K. (2011) 'The projected effect of risk factor reduction on Alzheimer's disease prevalence.' *Lancet Neurology 10*, 819–828.
28. Kivipelto, M., Helkala, E.L., Laakso, M.P. *et al.* (2001) 'Midlife vascular risk factors and Alzheimer's disease in later life: longitudinal, population based study.' *British Medical Journal 322*, 7300, 1447–1451.
29. Middleton, L.E. and Yaffe, K. (2009) 'Promising strategies for the prevention of dementia.' *Archives of Neurology 66*, 10, 1210–1215.
30. Eckert, G.P., Kirsch, C., Leutz, S. *et al.* (2003) 'Cholesterol modulates amyloid beta-peptide's membrane interactions.' *Pharmacopsychiatry 36*, Suppl. 2, S136–143.
31. Middleton, L.E. and Yaffe, K. (2009) 'Promising strategies for the prevention of dementia.' *Archives of Neurology 66*, 10, 1210–1215.
32. Rockwood, K., Kirkland, S., Hogan, D.B. *et al.* (2002) 'Use of lipid-lowering agents, indication bias, and the risk of dementia in community-dwelling elderly people.' *Archives of Neurology 59*, 2, 223–227.
33. Luchsinger, J.A., Tang, M.-X., Shea, S. *et al.* (2002) 'Caloric intake and the risk of Alzheimer's disease.' *Archives of Neurology 59*, 1258–1263.
34. Gustafson, D., Rothenberg, E., Blennow, K. *et al.* (2003) 'An 18-year follow-up of overweight and risk of Alzheimer disease.' *Archives of Internal Medicine 163*, 1524–1528.
35. Low, L.-F., Yap, M.H.W. and Brodaty, H. (2010) 'Will testing for apolipoprotein E assist in tailoring dementia risk reduction? A review.' *Neuroscience and Biobehavioral Reviews 34*, 408–437.
36. Barnes, D.E. and Yaffe, K. (2011) 'The projected effect of risk factor reduction on Alzheimer's disease prevalence.' *Lancet Neurology 10*, 819–828.
37. Kern, S., Skoog, I., Östling, S. *et al.* (2012) 'Does low-dose acetylsalicylic acid prevent cognitive decline in women with high cardiovascular risk? A 5-year follow-up of a non-demented population-based cohort of Swedish elderly women.' *BMJ Open*, e001288. doi:10.1136/bmjopen-2012-001288.
38. Newman, M.F., Kirchner, J.L., Phillips-Bute, B. *et al.* (2001) 'Longitudinal assessment of neurocognitive function after coronary-artery bypass surgery.' *The New England Journal of Medicine 344*, 6, 395–402.
39. Silbert, B.S., Scott, D.A., Evered, L.A. *et al.* (2007) 'Preexisting cognitive impairment in patients scheduled for elective coronary artery bypass graft surgery.' *Anesth Analg 104*, 1023–1028.
40. LeBlanc, E.S., Janowsky, J., Chan, B.K.S. *et al.* (2001) 'Hormone replacement therapy and cognition: systematic review and meta-analysis.' *JAMA 285*, 1489–1499.
41. Writing Group for the Women's Health Initiative Investigators (2002) 'Risks and benefits of estrogen plus progestin in healthy postmenopausal women: principal results from the Women's Health Initiative randomized controlled trial.' *JAMA 288*, 3, 321–333.

42. Vickers, M.R., MacLennan, A.H., Lawton, B. *et al.* (2007) 'Main morbidities recorded in the women's international study of long duration oestrogen after menopause (WISDOM): a randomised controlled trial of hormone replacement therapy in postmenopausal women.' *BMJ 335*, 7613, 239.

43. Shumaker, S.A., Legault, C., Kuller, L., *et al.* (2004) 'Conjugated equine estrogens and incidence of probable dementia and mild cognitive impairment in postmenopausal women: Women's Health Initiative Memory Study.' *JAMA 23*, 291, 24, 2947–2958.

44. Maki, P.M. and Henderson, V.W. (2012) 'Hormone therapy, dementia, and cognition: the Women's Health Initiative 10 years on.' *Climacteric 15*, 3, 256–262.

45. Vickers, M.R., MacLennan, A.H., Lawton, B. *et al.* (2007) 'Main morbidities recorded in the women's international study of long duration oestrogen after menopause (WISDOM): a randomised controlled trial of hormone replacement therapy in postmenopausal women.' *BMJ 335*, 7613, 239.

46. Gillett, M.J., Martins, R.N., Clarnette, R.M. *et al.* (2003) 'Relationship between testosterone, sex hormone binding globulin and plasma amyloid beta peptide 40 in older men with subjective memory loss or dementia.' *Journal of Alzheimer's Disease 5*, (4) 267–269.

47. in 't Veld B.A., Ruitenberg, A., Hofman, A. *et al.* (2001) 'Nonsteroidal antiinflammatory drugs and the risk of Alzheimer's disease.' *New England Journal of Medicine 345*, 21, 1515–1521.

48. Breitner, J.C., Baker, L.D., Montine, T.J., *et al.* (2011) 'Extended results of the Alzheimer's disease anti-inflammatory prevention trial.' *Alzheimer's & Dementia: The Journal of the Alzheimer's Association 7*, 4, 402–411.

49. Breitner, J.C., Baker, L.D., Montine, T.J., *et al.* (2011) 'Extended results of the Alzheimer's disease anti-inflammatory prevention trial.' *Alzheimer's & Dementia: The Journal of the Alzheimer's Association 7*, 4, 402–411.

50. Helmer, C., Letenneur, L., Rouch, I. *et al.* (2001) 'Occupation during life and risk of dementia in French elderly community residents.' *Journal of Neurology, Neurosurgery & Psychiatry 71*, 3, 303–309.

51. Tyas, S.L., Manfreda, J., Strain, L.A. *et al.* (2001) 'Risk factors for Alzheimer's disease: a population-based, longitudinal study in Manitoba, Canada.' *International Journal of Epidemiology 30*, 3, 590–597.

52. Hayden, K.M., Norton, M.C., Darcey, D. *et al.* (2010) 'Occupational exposure to pesticides increases the risk of incident AD: the Cache County Study.' *Neurology 74*, 1524–1530.

53. Smyth, K.A., Fritsch, T., Cook, T.B. *et al.* (2004) 'Worker functions and traits associated with occupations and the development of AD.' *Neurology 63*, 498–503.

54. Friedland, R.P., Fritsch, T., Smyth, K.A. *et al.* (2001) 'Patients with Alzheimer's disease have reduced activities in midlife compared with healthy control-group members.' *PNAS 98*, 3440–3445.

55. Andel, R., Crowe, M., Hahn, E.A. *et al.* (2012) Work-related stress may increase the risk of vascular dementia.' *Journal of the American Geriatrics Society 60*, 1, 60–67.

56. Baranov, D., Bickler, P.E., Crosby, G.J. *et al.* (2009) 'Consensus statement: first international workshop on anaesthetics and Alzheimer's disease.' *Anesth. Analg. 108*, 1627–1630.

57. Fong, T.G., Jones, R.N., Shi, P. *et al.* (2009) 'Delirium accelerates cognitive decline in Alzheimer disease.' *Neurology 72*, 18, 1570–1575.

58. Krogseth, M., Wyller, T.B., Engedal, K. and Juliebo, V. (2011) 'Delirium is an important predictor of incident dementia among elderly hip fracture patients.' *Dementia & Geriatric Cognitive Disorders 31*, 1, 63–70.

59. Inouye, S.K., Bogardus, S.T. Jr., Baker, D.I. *et al.* (2000) 'The Hospital Elder Life Programme: a model of care to prevent cognitive and functional decline in older hospitalised patients.' *Journal of the American Geriatrics Society 48*, 12, 1697–1706.

60. Winblad, B., Palmer, K., Kivipelto, M. *et al.* (2004) 'Mild cognitive impairment – beyond controversies, towards a consensus: report of the International Working Group on Mild Cognitive Impairment.' *Journal of Internal Medicine 256*, 240–246.

61. Petersen, R.C., Roberts, R.O., Knopman, D., *et al.* (2009) 'Mild cognitive impairment: ten years later.' *Archives of Neurology 66*, 1447–1455.

62. McKhann, G.M., Knopman, D.S., Chertkow, H. *et al.* (2011) 'The diagnosis of dementia due to Alzheimer's disease: recommendations from the National Institute on Aging–Alzheimer's Association workgroups on diagnostic guidelines for Alzheimer's disease.' *Alzheimer's & Dementia 7*, 263–269.

63. Barnes, D.E. and Yaffe, K. (2011) 'The projected effect of risk factor reduction on Alzheimer's disease prevalence.' *Lancet Neurology 10*, 819–828.

64. Barnes, D.E., Yaffe, K., Byers, A.L. *et al.* (2012) 'Midlife vs late-life depressive symptoms and risk of dementia. differential effects for alzheimer disease and vascular dementia.' *Archives of General Psychiatry 69*, 5, 493–498.

65. Barnes, D.E., Yaffe, K., Byers, A.L. *et al.* (2012) 'Midlife vs late-life depressive symptoms and risk of dementia. differential effects for alzheimer disease and vascular dementia.' *Archives of General Psychiatry 69*, 5, 493–498.

66. Brodaty, H., Luscombe, G., Peisah, C. *et al.* (2001) 'A 25-year longitudinal comparison study of the outcome of depression.' *Psychological Medicine 31*, 8, 1347–1359.

67. Barnes, D.E. and Yaffe, K. (2011) 'The projected effect of risk factor reduction on Alzheimer's disease prevalence.' *Lancet Neurology 10*, 819–828.

68. Billioti de Gage, S., Bégaud, B. and Bazin, F. *et al.* (2012) 'Benzodiazepine use and risk of dementia: prospective population based study.' *BMJ 345*, e6231. doi: 10.1136/bmj. e6231.

69. Draper, B., Pfaff, J., Pirkis, J. *et al.* (2008) 'The long-term effects of childhood abuse on the quality of life and health of older people: results from the Depression and Early Prevention of Suicide in General Practice Project.' *Journal of the American Geriatrics Society 56*, 262–271.

70. Yaffe, K., Vittinghoff, E., Lindquist, K., *et al.* (2010) 'Posttraumatic Stress Disorder and risk of dementia among US veterans.' *Archives of General Psychiatry 67*, 6, 608–613.

71. Qureshi, S., Kimbrell, T., Pyne, J., *et al.* (2010) 'Greater prevalence and incidence of dementia in older veterans with posttraumatic stress disorder.' *Journal of the American Geriatrics Society 58*, 9, 1627–1633.

72. Qureshi, S.U., Long, M.E., Bradshaw, M.R. *et al.* (2011) 'Does PTSD impair cognition beyond the effect of trauma?' *The Journal of Neuropsychiatry and Clinical Neurosciences 23*, 1, 16–28.

73. Chapman, M.R., Robinson, L.S. and Pinkner, J.S. *et al.* (2002) 'Role of Escherichia coli curli operons in directing amyloid fiber formation.' *Science 295*, 5556, 851–855.

74. DeKosky, S.T., Williamson, J.D., Fitzpatrick, A.L. *et al.* (2008) 'Ginkgo biloba for prevention of dementia: a randomized controlled trial.' *JAMA 300*, 2253–2262.

75. Vellas, B., Coley, N., Ousset, P.J. *et al.* (2012) 'Long-term use of standardised ginkgo biloba extract in this trial did not reduce the risk of progression to Alzheimer's disease compared with placebo.' *Lancet Neurology 11*, 10, 851–859.

Chapter 4

1. Weintraub, S. (2000) 'Neuropsychological assessment of mental state.' In M.M. Mesulam (ed.) *Principles of Behavioral and Cognitive Neurology*. Oxford: Oxford University Press.

2. US Department of Health and Human Services (2008) *Alzheimer's Disease: Unraveling the Mystery*. NIH Publication number: 08–3782, September.

3. Draper, B. (1999) 'The diagnosis and treatment of depression in dementia.' *Psychiatric Services 50*, 1151–1153.

4. Draper, B. (ed.) (2010) *The IPA Complete Guide to Behavioral and Psychological Symptoms of Dementia.* Chicago: International Psychogeriatric Association.

5. Draper, B. (ed.) (2010) *The IPA Complete Guide to Behavioral and Psychological Symptoms of Dementia.* Chicago: International Psychogeriatric Association.

6. US Department of Health and Human Services (2008) *Alzheimer's Disease: Unraveling the Mystery.* NIH Publication number: 08–3782, September.

7. Draper, B. (ed.) (2010) *The IPA Complete Guide to Behavioral and Psychological Symptoms of Dementia.* Chicago: International Psychogeriatric Association.

8. Draper, B. (1999) 'The diagnosis and treatment of depression in dementia.' *Psychiatric Services 50*, 1151–1153.

9. Draper, B., Brodaty, H., Low, L.-F. *et al.* (2002) 'Self destructive behaviours in nursing home residents.' *Journal of the American Geriatrics Society 50*, 354–358.

10. Mecocci, P., von Strauss, E., Cherubini, A. et al. (2005) 'Cognitive impairment is the major risk factor for development of geriatric syndromes during hospitalization: results from the GIFA Study.' *Dementia and Geriatric Cognitive Disorders 20*, 262–269.

Chapter 5

1. Alzheimer's Disease International (2009) *World Alzheimer Report 2009.* Edited by M. Prince and J. Jackson. Available at www.alz.co.uk/research/world-report, accessed on 8 December 2012.

2. Draper, B. (1991) 'Potentially Reversible Dementia – a review.' *Australian and New Zealand Journal of Psychiatry 25*, 506–18.

3. Lovestone, S. and McLoughlin, D.M. (2002) 'Protein aggregates and dementia: is there a common toxicity?' *Journal of Neurology, Neurosurgery and Psychiatry 72*, 2, 152–161.

4. US Department of Health and Human Services (2008) *Alzheimer's Disease: Unraveling the Mystery.* NIH Publication number: 08–3782, September.

5. US Department of Health and Human Services (2008) *Alzheimer's Disease: Unraveling the Mystery.* NIH Publication number: 08–3782, September.

6. Blessed, G., Tomlinson, B.E. and Roth, M. (1968) 'The association between quantitative measures of dementia and of senile change in the cerebral grey matter of elderly subjects.' *British Journal of Psychiatry 114*, 512, 797–811.

7. Tomlinson, B.E., Blessed, G. and Roth, M. (1970) 'Observations on the brains of demented old people.' *Journal of the Neurological Sciences 11*, 3, 205–242.

8. Katzman, R. (1976) Editorial: 'The prevalence and malignancy of Alzheimer disease: a major killer.' *Archives of Neurology 33*, 4, 217–218.

9. US Department of Health and Human Services (2008) *Alzheimer's Disease: Unraveling the Mystery.* NIH Publication number: 08–3782, September.

10. Lovestone, S. and McLoughlin, D.M. (2002) 'Protein aggregates and dementia: is there a common toxicity?' *Journal of Neurology, Neurosurgery and Psychiatry 72*, 2, 152–161.

11. US Department of Health and Human Services (2008) *Alzheimer's Disease: Unraveling the Mystery.* NIH Publication number: 08–3782, September.

12. US Department of Health and Human Services (2008) *Alzheimer's Disease: Unraveling the Mystery.* NIH Publication number: 08–3782, September.

13. Lovestone, S. (2000) 'Fleshing out the amyloid cascade hypothesis: the molecular biology of Alzheimer's disease.' *Dialogues in Clinical Neuroscience 2*, 2, 101–110.

14. Lovestone, S. (2000) 'Fleshing out the amyloid cascade hypothesis: the molecular biology of Alzheimer's disease.' *Dialogues in Clinical Neuroscience 2*, 2, 101–110.

15. Lovestone, S. (2000) 'Fleshing out the amyloid cascade hypothesis: the molecular biology of Alzheimer's disease.' *Dialogues in Clinical Neuroscience 2*, 2, 101–110.

16. US Department of Health and Human Services (2008) *Alzheimer's Disease: Unraveling the Mystery.* NIH Publication number: 08–3782, September.

17. US Department of Health and Human Services (2008) *Alzheimer's Disease: Unraveling the Mystery.* NIH Publication number: 08–3782, September.

18. Lovestone, S. (2000) 'Fleshing out the amyloid cascade hypothesis: the molecular biology of Alzheimer's disease.' *Dialogues in Clinical Neuroscience 2*, 2, 101–110.

19. Perry, E.K., Tomlinson, B.E., Blessed, G. *et al.* (1978) 'Correlation of cholinergic abnormalities with senile plaques and mental test scores in senile dementia.' *British Medical Journal 2*, 1457–1459.

20. Draper, B. (ed.) (2010) *The IPA Complete Guide to Behavioral and Psychological Symptoms of Dementia.* Chicago: International Psychogeriatric Association.

21. Gustafson, L. (2000) 'Historical Overview.' In E. Chiu, L. Gustafson, D. Ames and M.F. Folstein (eds) *Cerebrovascular Disease and Dementia.* London: Martin Dunitz Ltd.

22. Kirshner, H.S. (2009) 'Vascular dementia: a review of recent evidence for prevention and treatment.' *Current Neurology and Neuroscience Reports 9*, 437–442.

23. Brun, A. (2000) 'The Neuropathology of Vascular Dementia.' In E. Chiu, L. Gustafson, D. Ames and M.F. Folstein (eds) *Cerebrovascular Disease and Dementia.* London: Martin Dunitz Ltd.

24. Erkinjuntti, T. (2000) 'Classification and Criteria.' In E. Chiu, L. Gustafson, D. Ames and M.F. Folstein (eds) *Cerebrovascular Disease and Dementia.* London: Martin Dunitz Ltd.

25. Erkinjuntti, T. (2000) 'Classification and Criteria.' In E. Chiu, L. Gustafson, D. Ames and M.F. Folstein (eds) *Cerebrovascular Disease and Dementia.* London: Martin Dunitz Ltd.

26. Kirshner, H.S. (2009) 'Vascular dementia: a review of recent evidence for prevention and treatment.' *Current Neurology and Neuroscience Reports 9*, 437–442.

27. McKeith, I.G., Galasko, D., Kosaka, K. *et al.* (1996) 'Consensus guidelines for the clinical and pathologic diagnosis of dementia with Lewy bodies (DLB): report of the consortium on DLB international workshop.' *Neurology 47*, 1113–1124.

28. Alzheimer's Disease International (2009) *World Alzheimer Report 2009.* Edited by M. Prince and J. Jackson. Available at www.alz.co.uk/research/world-report, accessed on 8 December 2012.

29. McKeith, I.G., Galasko, D., Kosaka, K. *et al.* (1996) 'Consensus guidelines for the clinical and pathologic diagnosis of dementia with Lewy bodies (DLB): report of the consortium on DLB international workshop.' *Neurology 47*, 1113–1124.

30. McKeith, I.G., Galasko, D., Kosaka, K. *et al.* (1996) 'Consensus guidelines for the clinical and pathologic diagnosis of dementia with Lewy bodies (DLB): report of the consortium on DLB international workshop.' *Neurology 47*, 1113–24.

31. Lovestone, S. and McLoughlin, D.M. (2002) 'Protein aggregates and dementia: is there a common toxicity?' *Journal of Neurology, Neurosurgery and Psychiatry 72*, 2, 152–161.

32. McKeith, I., Del Ser, T., Spano, P. *et al.* (2000) 'Efficacy of rivastigmine in dementia with Lewy bodies: a randomised, double-blind, placebo-controlled international study.' *Lancet 16*, 356, 9247, 2031–2036.

33. Frontier – Frontotemporal Dementia Research Group (undated) 'What is frontotemporal dementia?' Available at www.ftdrg.org/caregivers/ftd/, accessed on 24 February 2010.

34. Rascovsky, K., Hodges, J.R., Knopman, D. *et al.* (2011) 'Sensitivity of revised diagnostic criteria for the behavioural variant of frontotemporal dementia.' *Brain 134* (pt9), 2456–2477.

35. Gorno-Tempini, M.L., Hillis, A.E., *et al.* (2011) 'Classification of primary progressive aphasia and its variants.' *Neurology 15*, 76, 11, 1006–1114.

36. Gorno-Tempini, M.L., Hillis, A.E., *et al.* (2011) 'Classification of primary progressive aphasia and its variants.' *Neurology 15*, 76, 11, 1006–1114.

37. Frontier – Frontotemporal Dementia Research Group (undated) 'What is frontotemporal dementia?' Available at www.ftdrg.org/caregivers/ftd/, accessed on 24 February 2010.

38. van Swieten, J.C., Rosso, S.M. and Heutink, P. (2010) 'MAPT-related disorders.' *GeneReviews.* Available at www.ncbi.nlm.nih.gov/books/NBK1505/, accessed on 29 December 2012.

39. Knight, R.S.G. and Will, R.G. (2004) 'Prion diseases.' *Journal of Neurology, Neurosurgery and Psychiatry 75* (Suppl I), i36–i42.

40. Lovestone, S. and McLoughlin, D.M. (2002) 'Protein aggregates and dementia: is there a common toxicity?' Journal of Neurology, Neurosurgery and Psychiatry 72, 2, 152–161.

41. Strömgren, E., Dalby, A., Dalby, M.A. and Ranheim, B. (1970) 'Cataract, deafness, cerebellar ataxia, psychosis and dementia – a new syndrome.' *Acta Neurol Scand 46*, Suppl 43, 261+.

42. Draper, B. (1991) 'Potentially Reversible Dementia – a review.' *Australian and New Zealand Journal of Psychiatry 25*, 506–518.

43. Draper, B. (1991) 'Potentially Reversible Dementia – a review.' *Australian and New Zealand Journal of Psychiatry 25*, 506–518.

44. Ridley, N., Draper, B. and Withall, A. (2013) 'Alcohol-related dementia: an update of the evidence.' *Alzheimer's Research & Therapy 5*, 3. Available at: http://alzres.com/content/5/1/3.

45. Sacktor, N., McDermott, M.P., Marder, K. *et al.* (2002) 'HIV-associated cognitive impairment before and after the advent of combination therapy.' *Journal of Neurovirology 8*, 136–142.

46. Welch, K. and Morse, A. (2002) 'The clinical profile of end-stage AIDS in the era of highly active antiretroviral therapy.' *AIDS Patient Care & Standards 16*, 75–81.

47. Wright, E.J. (2009) 'Neurological disease: the effects of HIV and antiretroviral therapy and the implications for early antiretroviral therapy initiation.' *Current Opinion in HIV & AIDS 4*, 5, 447–452.

Chapter 6

1. Hodkinson, H.M. (1972) 'Evaluation of a mental test score for assessment of mental impairment in the elderly.' *Age and Ageing 1*, 4, 233–238.

2. Storey, J., Rowland, J., Basic, D. *et al.* (2004) 'The Rowland Universal Dementia Assessment Scale (RUDAS): a multicultural cognitive assessment scale.' *International Psychogeriatrics 16*, 1, 13–31.

3. Folstein, M.F., Folstein, S.E. and McHugh, P.R. (1975) '"Mini-mental state": a practical method for grading the cognitive state of patients for the clinician.' *Journal of Psychiatric Research 12*, 3, 189–198.

4. Brodaty, H., Pond, D., Kemp, N.M. *et al.* (2002) 'The GPCOG: a new screening test for dementia designed for general practice.' *Journal of the American Geriatrics Society 50*, 530–534.

5. Hodkinson, H.M. (1972) 'Evaluation of a mental test score for assessment of mental impairment in the elderly.' *Age and Ageing 1*, 4, 233–238.

6. Folstein, M.F., Folstein, S.E. and McHugh, P.R. (1975) '"Mini-mental state": a practical method for grading the cognitive state of patients for the clinician.' *Journal of Psychiatric Research 12*, 3, 189–198.

7. Storey, J., Rowland, J., Basic, D. *et al.* (2004) 'The Rowland Universal Dementia Assessment Scale (RUDAS): a multicultural cognitive assessment scale.' *International Psychogeriatrics 16*, 1, 13–31.

8. Brodaty, H., Pond, D., Kemp, N.M. *et al.* (2002) 'The GPCOG: a new screening test for dementia designed for general practice.' *Journal of the American Geriatrics Society 50*, 530–534.

9. American Psychiatric Association Work Group on Alzheimer's Disease and other Dementias (2007) 'American Psychiatric Association practice guideline for the treatment of patients with Alzheimer's disease and other dementias: second edition.' *American Journal of Psychiatry 164* (12 Suppl.), 5–56.

10. Draper, B. (1999) 'The diagnosis and treatment of depression in dementia.' *Psychiatric Services 50*, 1151–1153.

11. Kiloh, L. (1961) 'Pseudo-dementia.' *Acta Psychiatrica Scandinavica 37*, 336–351.

12. Draper, B. (1999) 'The diagnosis and treatment of depression in dementia.' *Psychiatric Services 50*, 1151–1153.

13. Draper, B. (1991) 'Potentially Reversible Dementia – a review.' *Australian and New Zealand Journal of Psychiatry 25*, 506–518.

14. Winblad, B., Palmer, K., Kivipelto, M. *et al.* (2004) 'Mild cognitive impairment – beyond controversies, towards a consensus: report of the International Working Group on Mild Cognitive Impairment.' *Journal of Internal Medicine 256*, 240–246.

15. Ridley, N., Draper, B. and Withall, A. (2013) 'Alcohol-related dementia: an update of the evidence.' *Alzheimer's Research & Therapy* 5, 3. Available at: http://alzres.com/contnet/5/1/3.

16. McKhann, G.M., Knopman, D.S., Chertkow, H. *et al.* (2011) 'The diagnosis of dementia due to Alzheimer's disease: recommendations from the National Institute on Aging–Alzheimer's Association workgroups on diagnostic guidelines for Alzheimer's disease.' *Alzheimer's & Dementia 7*, 263–269.

17. McKhann, G.M., Knopman, D.S., Chertkow, H. *et al.* (2011) 'The diagnosis of dementia due to Alzheimer's disease: recommendations from the National Institute on Aging–Alzheimer's Association workgroups on diagnostic guidelines for Alzheimer's disease.' *Alzheimer's & Dementia 7*, 263–269.

18. Draper, B., Peisah, C., Snowdon, J. and Brodaty, H. (2010) 'Early dementia diagnosis and the risk of suicide and euthanasia.' *Alzheimer's & Dementia 6*, 75–82.

Chapter 7

1. American Psychiatric Association Work Group on Alzheimer's Disease and other Dementias (2007) 'American Psychiatric Association practice guideline for the treatment of patients with Alzheimer's disease and other dementias: second edition.' *American Journal of Psychiatry 164* (12 Suppl.), 5–56.

2. National Institute for Health and Clinical Excellence (2011) 'NICE technology appraisal guidance 217: donepezil, galantamine, rivastigmine and memantine for the treatment of Alzheimer's disease (review of NICE technology appraisal guidance 111).' Available at www.nice.org.uk/TA217, accessed on 31 December 2012.

3. Erkinjuntti, T., Kurz, A., Gauthier, S. *et al.* (2002) 'Efficacy of galantamine in probable vascular dementia and Alzheimer's disease combined with cerebrovascular disease: a randomised trial.' *Lancet 359*, 1283–1290.

4. American Psychiatric Association Work Group on Alzheimer's Disease and other Dementias (2007) 'American Psychiatric Association practice guideline for the treatment of patients with Alzheimer's disease and other dementias: second edition.' *American Journal of Psychiatry 164* (12 Suppl.), 5–56.

5. National Institute for Health and Clinical Excellence (2011) 'NICE technology appraisal guidance 217: donepezil, galantamine, rivastigmine and memantine for the treatment of Alzheimer's disease (review of NICE technology appraisal guidance 111).' Available at www.nice.org.uk/TA217, accessed on 31 December 2012.

6. Schwartz, L.M. and Woloshin, S. (2012) 'How the FDA forgot the evidence: the case of donepezil 23 mg.' *BMJ 344*, e1086.

7. American Psychiatric Association Work Group on Alzheimer's Disease and other Dementias (2007) 'American Psychiatric Association practice guideline for the treatment of patients with Alzheimer's disease and other dementias: second edition.' *American Journal of Psychiatry 164* (12 Suppl.), 5–56.

8. National Institute for Health and Clinical Excellence (2011) 'NICE technology appraisal guidance 217: donepezil, galantamine, rivastigmine and memantine for the treatment of Alzheimer's disease (review of NICE technology appraisal guidance 111).' Available at www.nice.org.uk/TA217, accessed on 31 December 2012.

9. National Institute for Health and Clinical Excellence (2011) 'NICE technology appraisal guidance 217: donepezil, galantamine, rivastigmine and memantine for the treatment of Alzheimer's disease (review of NICE technology appraisal guidance 111).' Available at www.nice.org.uk/TA217, accessed on 31 December 2012.

10. British Columbia Ministry of Health (2011) 'Alzheimer's Drug Therapy Initiative.' Available at: www.health.gov.bc.ca/pharmacare/adti/index.html, accessed on 31 December 2012.

11. Howard, R., McShane, R., Lindesay, J. *et al.* (2012) 'Donepezil and memantine for moderate-to-severe Alzheimer's disease.' *New England Journal of Medicine 366*, 893–903.

12. Department of Health and Ageing (2012) Post Market Review. Pharmaceutical Benefits Scheme anti-dementia medicines to treat Alzheimer Disease. Report to the Pharmaceutical Benefits Advisory Committee, October 2012. Available at www.pbs.gov.au/info/reviews/anti-dementia-report, accessed on 31 December 2012.

13. National Institute for Health and Clinical Excellence (2011) 'NICE technology appraisal guidance 217: donepezil, galantamine, rivastigmine and memantine for the treatment of Alzheimer's disease (review of NICE technology appraisal guidance 111).' Available at www.nice.org.uk/TA217, accessed on 31 December 2012.

14. American Psychiatric Association Work Group on Alzheimer's Disease and other Dementias (2007) 'American Psychiatric Association practice guideline for the treatment of patients with Alzheimer's disease and other dementias: second edition.' *American Journal of Psychiatry 164* (12 Suppl.), 5–56.

15. Howard, R., McShane, R., Lindesay, J. *et al.* (2012) 'Donepezil and memantine for moderate-to-severe Alzheimer's disease.' *New England Journal of Medicine 366*, 893–903.

16. Sijben, J.W.C., de Wilde, M.C., Wieggers, R., Groenendijk, M. and Kamphuis, P.J.G.H. (2011) 'A multi nutrient concept to enhance synapse formation and function: science behind a medical food for Alzheimer's disease.' OCL 18, 267–270. doi: 10.1684/ocl.2011.0410.

17. Scheltens, P., Kamphuis, P.J., Verhey, F.R. et al. (January 2010) 'Efficacy of a medical food in mild Alzheimer's disease: a randomized, controlled trial.' *Alzheimer's & Dementia 6*, 1, 1–10.e1. doi:10.1016/j.jalz.2009.10.003. PMID 20129316.

18. American Psychiatric Association Work Group on Alzheimer's Disease and other Dementias (2007) 'American Psychiatric Association practice guideline for the treatment of patients with Alzheimer's disease and other dementias: second edition.' *American Journal of Psychiatry 164* (12 Suppl.), 5–56.

19. American Psychiatric Association Work Group on Alzheimer's Disease and other Dementias (2007) 'American Psychiatric Association practice guideline for the treatment of patients with Alzheimer's disease and other dementias: second edition.' *American Journal of Psychiatry 164* (12 Suppl.), 5–56.

20. American Psychiatric Association Work Group on Alzheimer's Disease and other Dementias (2007) 'American Psychiatric Association practice guideline for the treatment of patients with Alzheimer's disease and other dementias: second edition.' *American Journal of Psychiatry 164* (12 Suppl.), 5–56.

21. Hao, Z., Liu, M., Liu, Z. *et al.* (2011) 'Huperzine A for vascular dementia.' doi: 10.1002/14651858.CD007365.pub2.

22. Li, J., Wu, H.M., Zhou, R.L. *et al.* (2009) 'Huperzine A for Alzheimer's disease.' doi: 10.1002/14651858.CD005592.pub2.

23. Alzheimer's Association. 'Alternative treatments.' Available at www.alz.org/alzheimers_disease_alternative_treatments.asp, accessed on 31 December 2012.

24. American Psychiatric Association Work Group on Alzheimer's Disease and other Dementias (2007) 'American Psychiatric Association practice guideline for the treatment of patients with Alzheimer's disease and other dementias: second edition.' *American Journal of Psychiatry 164* (12 Suppl.), 5–56.

25. Alzheimer's Association. 'Alternative treatments.' Available at www.alz.org/alzheimers_disease_alternative_treatments.asp, accessed on 31 December 2012.

26. Sabbagh, M.N. (2009) 'Drug developments for Alzheimer's disease: where are we now and where are we headed.' *The American Journal of Geriatric Pharmacotherapy 7,* 167–185.

27. Draper, B. (ed.) (2010) The IPA Complete Guide to Behavioral and Psychological Symptoms of Dementia. Chicago: International Psychogeriatric Association.

28. Draper, B., Brodaty, H., Low, L.-F. *et al.* (2001) 'Use of psychotropics in Sydney nursing homes: associations with psychosis, depression and behavioural disturbances.' *International Psychogeriatrics 13,* 107–120.

29. Draper, B., Brodaty, H., Low, L.-F. *et al.* (2001) 'Use of psychotropics in Sydney nursing homes: associations with psychosis, depression and behavioural disturbances.' *International Psychogeriatrics 13,* 107–120.

30. Rendina, N., Brodaty, H., Draper, B. *et al.* (2009) 'Substitute consent for nursing home residents prescribed psychotropic medication.' *International Psychogeriatrics 24,* 226–231.

31. American Psychiatric Association Work Group on Alzheimer's Disease and other Dementias (2007) 'American Psychiatric Association practice guideline for the treatment of patients with Alzheimer's disease and other dementias: second edition.' *American Journal of Psychiatry 164* (12 Suppl.), 5–56.

32. Schneider, L.S., Tariot, P.N., Dagerman, K.S. *et al.* (2006) 'Effectiveness of atypical antipsychotic drugs in patients with Alzheimer's disease.' *New England Journal of Medicine 355,* 1525–1538.

33. Committee on Safety of Medicines Pharmacovigilance Working Party Public Assessment Report (2007) 'Antipsychotics and risk of cerebrovascular accident.' www.mhra.gov.uk/Safetyinformation/Generalsafetyinformationandadvice/Product-specificinformationandadvice/Product-specificinformationandadvice-A-F/Antipsychoticdrugs/index.htm, accessed on 31 December 2012.

34. Food and Drug Administration (2005) 'Deaths with antipsychotics in elderly patients with behavioural disturbances.' Available at www.fda.gov/Drugs/DrugSafety/PostmarketDrugSafetyInformationforPatientsandProviders/DrugSafetyInformationforHeathcareProfessionals/PublicHealthAdvisories/ucm053171.htm, accessed on 31 December 2012.

35. Schneider, L.S., Tariot, P.N., Dagerman, K.S. *et al.* (2006) 'Effectiveness of atypical antipsychotic drugs in patients with Alzheimer's disease.' *New England Journal of Medicine 355,* 1525–1538.

36. NPS News (2011) 'Balancing benefits and harms of antipsychotic therapy.' Available at www.nps.org.au/publications/health-professional/nps-news/2011/balancing-benefits-harms-of-antipsychotic-therapy, accessed on 31 December 2012.

37. NPS News (2011) 'Balancing benefits and harms of antipsychotic therapy.' Available at www.nps.org.au/publications/health-professional/nps-news/2011/balancing-benefits-harms-of-antipsychotic-therapy, accessed on 31 December 2012.

38. Ballard, C., Hanney, M.L., Theodoulou, M. *et al.* (2009) 'The dementia antipsychotic withdrawal trial (DART-AD): long-term follow-up of a randomised placebo-controlled trial.' *Lancet Neurology 8,* 2, 151–157.

39. Banerjee, S., Hellier, J., Dewey, M. *et al.* (2011) 'Sertraline or mirtazapine for depression in dementia (HTA-SADD): a randomised, multicentre, double-blind, placebo-controlled trial.' *Lancet 378*, 403–11.

40. Rosenberg, P.B., Drye, L.T., Martin, B.K. *et al.* (2010) 'Sertraline for the treatment of depression in Alzheimer disease.' American Journal of Geriatric Psychiatry 18, 2, 136–145.

41. Draper, B. (1999) 'The diagnosis and treatment of depression in dementia.' *Psychiatric Services 50*, 1151–1153.

42. Thompson, S., Herrmann, N., Rapoport, M.J. and Lanctot, K.L. (2007) 'Efficacy and safety of antidepressants for treatment of depression in Alzheimer's disease: a meta-analysis.' *Canadian Journal of Psychiatry 52*, 248–255.

43. American Psychiatric Association Work Group on Alzheimer's Disease and other Dementias (2007) 'American Psychiatric Association practice guideline for the treatment of patients with Alzheimer's disease and other dementias: second edition.' *American Journal of Psychiatry 164* (12 Suppl.), 5–56.

44. American Psychiatric Association Work Group on Alzheimer's Disease and other Dementias (2007) 'American Psychiatric Association practice guideline for the treatment of patients with Alzheimer's disease and other dementias: second edition.' *American Journal of Psychiatry 164* (12 Suppl.), 5–56.

45. Husebo, B.S., Ballard, C., Sandvik, R. *et al.* (2011) 'Efficacy of treating pain to reduce behavioural disturbances in residents of nursing homes with dementia: cluster randomised clinical trial.' *BMJ 343*, d4065.

46. Kurrle, S, Brodaty, H. and Hogarth, R. (2012) *Physical Comorbidities of Dementia.* Cambridge: Cambridge University Press.

Chapter 8

1. Kitwood, T. (1993) 'Person and process in dementia.' *International Journal of Geriatric Psychiatry 8*, 541–545.

2. Chenoweth, L., King, M.T., Jeon, Y.H. *et al.* (2009) 'Caring for Aged Dementia Care Resident Study (CADRES) of person-centred care, dementia-care mapping, and usual care in dementia: a cluster-randomised trial.' *Lancet Neurology 8*, 4, 317–325.

3. Draper, B., Peisah, C., Snowdon, J. and Brodaty, H. (2010) 'Early dementia diagnosis and the risk of suicide and euthanasia.' *Alzheimer's & Dementia 6*, 75–82.

4. Kitwood, T. (1993) 'Person and process in dementia.' *International Journal of Geriatric Psychiatry 8*, 541–545.

5. Kitwood, T. (1993) 'Person and process in dementia.' *International Journal of Geriatric Psychiatry 8*, 541–545.

6. Clare, L. and Woods, R.T. (2008) 'Cognitive rehabilitation and cognitive training for early-stage Alzheimer's disease and vascular dementia.' *Cochrane Database of Systematic Reviews 4*, CD003260.

7. Dementia Collaborative Research Centre. 'Brain Training Laboratory.' Available at: www.dementia.unsw.edu.au/index.php?option=com_dcrc&view=dcrc&layout=project&Itemid=101&research_topic=0&researcher=0&research_type=0&year=0&population=0&centre=0&keywords=&searchtype=&pid=68&search=true, accessed on 30 March 2013.

8. Woods, B., Aguirre, E., Spector, A. and Orrell, M. (2012) 'Cognitive stimulation to improve cognitive functioning in people with dementia.' Cochrane Database of Systematic Reviews Issue 2. Art. No.: CD005562. DOI: 10.1002/14651858.CD005562.pub2.

9. National Institute for Health and Clinical Excellence (2006) 'Dementia: supporting people with dementia and their carers in health and social care.' NICE Clinical Guideline 42, November. Available at www.nice.org.uk/guidance/cg42, accessed on 31 December 2012.

10. Prince, M., Bryce, R. and Ferri, C. (2011) 'World Alzheimer report: the benefits of early diagnosis and intervention.' *Alzheimer's Disease International.* Available at www.alz.co.uk/worldreport2011, accessed on 31 December 2012.

11. Orrell, M., Woods, B. and Spector, A. (2012) 'Should we use individual cognitive stimulation therapy to improve cognitive function in people with dementia?' *BMJ 344*, e633. doi: 10.1136/bmj.e633.

12. Jones, G. (1997) 'A review of Feil's validation method for communicating with and caring for dementia sufferers.' *Current Opinion in Psychiatry 10*, 326–332.

13. Jones, G. (1997) 'A review of Feil's validation method for communicating with and caring for dementia sufferers.' *Current Opinion in Psychiatry 10*, 326–332.

14. Neal, M., Barton Wright, P. (2003) 'Validation therapy for dementia.' *Cochrane Database of Systematic Reviews, Issue 3.* Art. No.: CD001394. DOI: 10.1002/14651858.CD001394.

15. Livingston, G., Johnston, K., Katona, C. *et al.* (2005). 'Systematic review of psychological approaches to the management of neuropsychiatric symptoms of dementia.' *American Journal of Psychiatry 162*, 11, 1996–2021.

16. Livingston, G., Johnston, K., Katona, C. *et al.* (2005). 'Systematic review of psychological approaches to the management of neuropsychiatric symptoms of dementia.' *American Journal of Psychiatry 162*, 11, 1996–2021.

17. Woods, B., Spector, A.E., Jones, C.A. *et al.* (2005) 'Reminiscence therapy for dementia.' Cochrane Database of Systematic Reviews, Issue 2. Art. No.: CD001120. DOI: 10.1002/14651858.CD001120.pub2.

18. Livingston, G., Johnston, K., Katona, C. *et al.* (2005). 'Systematic review of psychological approaches to the management of neuropsychiatric symptoms of dementia.' *American Journal of Psychiatry 162*, 11, 1996–2021.

19. Woods, B., Spector, A.E., Jones, C.A. *et al.* (2005) 'Reminiscence therapy for dementia.' Cochrane Database of Systematic Reviews, Issue 2. Art. No.: CD001120. DOI: 10.1002/14651858.CD001120.pub2.

20. Rands, G. (1999) 'Review: reality orientation improves cognitive functioning and behaviour in dementia.' Evidence-based Mental Health. Available at http://ebmh.bmj.com/content/2/1/17, accessed on 31 December 2012.

21. Rands, G. (1999) 'Review: reality orientation improves cognitive functioning and behaviour in dementia.' Evidence-based Mental Health. Available at http://ebmh.bmj.com/content/2/1/17, accessed on 31 December 2012.

22. Spector, A., Orrell, M., Davies, S. and Woods, B. (2007) WITHDRAWN: 'Reality orientation for dementia.' *Cochrane Database Systematic Reviews 18*, 3, CD001119.

23. O'Connor, D., Ames, D., Gardner, B. and King, M. (2009) 'Psychosocial treatments of behavior symptoms in dementia: a systematic review of reports meeting quality standards.' *International Psychogeriatrics 21*, 225–240.

24. O'Connor, D., Ames, D., Gardner, B. and King, M. (2009) 'Psychosocial treatments of behavior symptoms in dementia: a systematic review of reports meeting quality standards.' *International Psychogeriatrics 21*, 225–240.

25. O'Connor, D., Ames, D., Gardner, B. and King, M. (2009) 'Psychosocial treatments of behavior symptoms in dementia: a systematic review of reports meeting quality standards.' *International Psychogeriatrics 21*, 225–240.

26. O'Connor, D., Ames, D., Gardner, B. and King, M. (2009) 'Psychosocial treatments of behavior symptoms in dementia: a systematic review of reports meeting quality standards.' *International Psychogeriatrics 21*, 225–240.

27. Bird, M., Alexopoulos, P. and Adamowicz, J. (1995) 'Success and failure in five case studies: use of cued recall to ameliorate behaviour problems in senile dementia.' International *Journal of Geriatric Psychiatry 10*, 305–311.

28. Draper, B., Turner, J., McMinn, B. *et al.* (2003) 'Treatment outcomes of nursing home residents with vocally disruptive behaviour.' *Australasian Journal on Ageing 22,* 81–85.

29. O'Connor, D., Ames, D., Gardner, B. and King, M. (2009) 'Psychosocial treatments of behavior symptoms in dementia: a systematic review of reports meeting quality standards.' *International Psychogeriatrics 21,* 225–240.

30. Forbes, D., Culum, I., Lischka, A.R. *et al.* (2009) 'Light therapy for managing cognitive, sleep, functional, behavioural, or psychiatric disturbances in dementia.' Cochrane Database of Systematic Reviews, Issue 4. Art. No.: CD003946. DOI: 10.1002/14651858. CD003946.pub3.

31. Chung, J.C.C. and Lai, C.K.Y. (2002) 'Snoezelen for dementia.' *Cochrane Database of Systematic Reviews,* Issue 4. Art. No.: CD003152. DOI: 10.1002/14651858.CD003152.

Chapter 9

1. Brodaty, H., Green, A. and Low, L.-F. (2005) 'Family Carers for People with Dementia.' In A. Burns, J. O'Brien and D. Ames (eds) *Dementia* (Third Edition). London: Hodder Arnold.

2. Mace, N. and Rabins, P. (1999) *The 36-Hour Day: A Family Guide to Caring for Persons with Alzheimer's Disease, Related Dementing Illnesses, and Memory Loss in Later Life* (Third Edition). Baltimore: Johns Hopkins University Press.

3. Liddell, M.B., Lovestone, S. and Owen, M.J. (2001) 'Genetic risk of Alzheimer's disease: advising relatives.' *British Journal of Psychiatry 178,* 7–11.

4. American Psychiatric Association Work Group on Alzheimer's Disease and other Dementias (2007) 'American Psychiatric Association practice guideline for the treatment of patients with Alzheimer's disease and other dementias: second edition.' *American Journal of Psychiatry 164* (12 Suppl.), 5–56.

5. Draper, B. (2012) 'An early warning.' *Australian Doctor,* 9 November, 29–30.

6. Richardson, H.H. (1982) *The Fortunes of Richard Mahony.* Ringwood, Victoria: Penguin Books Australia (originally William Heinemann Ltd, 1930).

7. Draper, B. (2009) 'Richard Mahony: the misfortunes of younger onset dementia.' *Medical Journal of Australia 190,* 94–95.

8. Alzheimer's Australia (undated) 'Younger onset dementia.' Available at www.fightdementia. org.au/services/younger-onset-dementia.aspx, accessed on 31 December 2012.

9. Alzheimer's Association (undated) 'Younger/early onset Alzheimer's and dementia.' Available at www.alz.org/alzheimers_disease_early_onset.asp, accessed on 31 December 2012.

10. Liddell, M.B., Lovestone, S. and Owen, M.J. (2001) 'Genetic risk of Alzheimer's disease: advising relatives.' *British Journal of Psychiatry 178,* 7–11.

11. The Inspired Study (2012) Available at www.inspiredstudy.org, accessed on 31 December 2012.

12. Brodaty, H., Green, A. and Low, L.-F. (2005) 'Family Carers for People with Dementia.' In A. Burns, J. O'Brien and D. Ames (eds) *Dementia* (Third Edition). London: Hodder Arnold.

13. Brodaty, H., Green, A. and Low, L.-F. (2005) 'Family Carers for People with Dementia.' In A. Burns, J. O'Brien and D. Ames (eds) *Dementia* (Third Edition). London: Hodder Arnold.

14. Mace, N. and Rabins, P. (1999) *The 36-Hour Day: A Family Guide to Caring for Persons with Alzheimer's Disease, Related Dementing Illnesses, and Memory Loss in Later Life* (Third Edition). Baltimore: Johns Hopkins University Press.

15. Cooney, C. and Howard, R. (1995) 'Abuse of patients with dementia by carers – out of sight but not out of mind.' *International Journal of Geriatric Psychiatry 10,* 735–741.

16. Cooney, C. and Howard, R. (1995) 'Abuse of patients with dementia by carers – out of sight but not out of mind.' *International Journal of Geriatric Psychiatry 10,* 735–741.

17. Cooney, C. and Howard, R. (1995) 'Abuse of patients with dementia by carers – out of sight but not out of mind.' *International Journal of Geriatric Psychiatry 10,* 735–741.

18. Brodaty, H., Green, A. and Low, L.-F. (2005) 'Family Carers for People with Dementia.' In A. Burns, J. O'Brien and D. Ames (eds) Dementia (Third Edition). London: Hodder Arnold.

19. Mace, N. and Rabins, P. (1999) *The 36-Hour Day: A Family Guide to Caring for Persons with Alzheimer's Disease, Related Dementing Illnesses, and Memory Loss in Later Life* (Third Edition). Baltimore: Johns Hopkins University Press.

20. Franzen, J. (2001) *The Corrections*. London: Fourth Estate.

21. Franzen, J. (2002) 'Into the abyss.' *Sydney Morning Herald Good Weekend*, 11 May, 45–54.

22. Brodaty, H., Green, A. and Low, L.-F. (2005) 'Family Carers for People with Dementia.' In A. Burns, J. O'Brien and D. Ames (eds) *Dementia* (Third Edition). London: Hodder Arnold.

23. Morris, R.G., Woods, R.T., Davies, K.S. *et al.* (1991) 'Gender differences in carers of dementia sufferers.' *British Journal of Psychiatry 158*, Supplement 10, 69–74.

24. Gutmann, D. (1990) 'Psychological development and pathology in later adulthood.' In R. Nemiroff and C. Colarusso (eds) *New Dimensions in Adult Development*. New York: Basic Books.

25. Brodaty, H., Gresham, M. and Luscombe, G. (1997) 'The Prince Henry Hospital Dementia Caregivers Training Programme.' *International Journal of Geriatric Psychiatry 12*, 183–192.

26. Parker, D., Mills, S. and Abbey, J. (2008) 'Effectiveness of interventions that assist caregivers to support people with dementia living in the community: a systematic review.' *International Journal of Evidence Based Healthcare 6*, 2, 137–172.

Chapter 10

1. Thane, P. (2009) 'Memorandum submitted to the House of Commons' Health Committee Inquiry: Social Care.' Available at www.historyandpolicy.org/docs/thane_social_care.pdf, accessed on 31 December 2012.

2. Bookman, A. and Kimbrel, D. (2011) 'Families and elder care in the twenty-first century.' *The Future of Children 21*, 2, 117–140.

3. Audit Commission for Local Authorities in England and Wales (1986) *Making a Reality of Community Care*. London: HMSO.

4. Audit Commission for Local Authorities in England and Wales (1992) Community Care: Managing the Cascade of Change. Available at www.audit-commission.gov.uk/subwebs/publications/studies/studyPDF/1053.pdf, accessed on 31 December 2012.

5. Langan, M. (1990) 'Community care in the 90s: the community care White Paper "Caring for People".' *Critical Social Policy 29*, 58–70.

6. Thane, P. (2009) 'Memorandum submitted to the House of Commons' Health Committee Inquiry: Social Care.' Available at www.historyandpolicy.org/docs/thane_social_care.pdf, accessed on 31 December 2012.

7. Langan, M. (1990) 'Community care in the 90s: the community care White Paper "Caring for People".' *Critical Social Policy 29*, 58–70.

8. Samuel, M. (2010) 'Community Care's exclusive survey of views on the dementia strategy.' Available at www.communitycare.co.uk/Articles/25/03/2010/114121/community-cares-exclusive-survey-of-views-on-the-dementia-strategy.htm, accessed on 31 December 2012.

9. House of Commons All-Party Parliamentary Group on Dementia (2012) 'Unlocking diagnosis: the key to improving the lives of people with dementia.' July 2012. Available at http://alzheimers.org.uk/site/scripts/download_info.php?downloadID=873, accessed on 31 December 2012.

10. Bookman, A. and Kimbrel, D. (2011) 'Families and elder care in the twenty-first century.' *The Future of Children 21*, 2, 117–140.

11. Bookman, A. and Kimbrel, D. (2011) 'Families and elder care in the twenty-first century.' *The Future of Children 21*, 2, 117–140.

12. Eng, C., Pedulla, J., Eleazer, G.P. *et al.* (1997) 'Programme of All-inclusive Care for the Elderly (PACE): an innovative model of integrated geriatric care and financing.' *Journal of the American Geriatrics Society 45*, 2, 223–232.

13. Bookman, A. and Kimbrel, D. (2011) 'Families and elder care in the twenty-first century.' *The Future of Children 21*, 2, 117–140.

14. Department of Community Services and Health (1986) *Nursing Homes and Hostels Review.* Canberra: Australian Government Publishing Service.

15. Howe, A.L. (1997) 'From states of confusion to a National Action Plan for Dementia Care: the development of policies for dementia care in Australia.' *International Journal of Geriatric Psychiatry 12*, 165–172.

16. Patient.co.uk. 'Community care.' Available at: www.patient.co.uk/doctor/Community-Care.htm, accessed on 1 April 2013.

17. Citizens Advice Bureau. 'Community care.' Available at: www.adviceguide.org.uk/england/relationships_e/relationships_looking_after_people_e/community_care.htm, accessed on 1 April 2013.

18. Centers for Medicare and Medicaid Services (2008) 'Quick facts about Programs of All-inclusive Care for the Elderly (PACE).' Available at: www.cms.gov/Medicare/Health-Plans/pace/downloads/externalfactsheet.pdf, accessed on 1 April 2013.

19. Centers for Medicare and Medicaid Services (2008) 'Quick facts about Programs of All-inclusive Care for the Elderly (PACE).' Available at: www.cms.gov/Medicare/Health-Plans/pace/downloads/externalfactsheet.pdf, accessed on 1 April 2013.

20. Lee, H. and Cameron, M.H. (2004) 'Respite care for people with dementia and their carers.' Cochrane Database of Systematic Reviews, Issue 1. Art. No.: CD004396. doi: 10.1002/14651858.CD004396.pub2.

Chapter 11

1. Department of Health and Ageing. 'Help with aged care homes.' Available at www.agedcareaustralia.gov.au/internet/agedcare/publishing.nsf/Content/help+with+aged+care+homes, accessed on 31 December 2012.

2. Department of Health and Ageing (2009) Aged Care Funding Instrument (ACFI). Available at www.health.gov.au/acfi, accessed on 31 December 2012.

3. Brodaty, H., Draper, B. and Low, L.-F. (2003) 'Nursing home staff attitudes towards residents, strain related to dementia care and satisfaction with work.' *Journal of Advanced Nursing 44*, 6, 583–590.

4. Fleming, R., Crookes, P. and Shum, S. (2008) 'A review of the empirical literature on the design of physical environments for people with dementia.' Primary Dementia Collaborative Research Centre. Available at www.dementia.unsw.edu.au/DCRCweb.nsf/page/TechDesign, accessed on 5 April 2010.

5. Morley, J.E. and Flaherty, J.H. (2002) 'Putting the "home" back in nursing home.' *Journal of Gerontology: Medical Sciences 57A*, M419–421.

6. Baker, N.L., Cook, M.N., Arrighi, H.M. and Bullock, R. (2010) 'Hip fracture risk and subsequent mortality among Alzheimer's disease patients in the UK, 1988–2007.' *Age and Ageing.* doi: 10.1093/ageing/afq146.

7. Australian Institute of Health and Welfare (2009) *Residential Aged Care in Australia 2007–2008: A Statistical Overview. Aged Care Statistic Series 28.* Cat. no. AGE 58. Canberra: AIHW.

8. US Department of Health and Human Services (2011) *Your Guide to Choosing a Nursing Home.* Available at www.medicare.gov/Pubs/pdf/02174.pdf, accessed on 31 December 2012.

9. US Department of Health and Human Services (2011) *Your Guide to Choosing a Nursing Home.* Available at www.medicare.gov/Pubs/pdf/02174.pdf, accessed on 31 December 2012.

10. Office of Fair Trading (2005) *Care Homes for Older People in the UK. A Market Study May 2005*. Available at www.oft.gov.uk/shared_oft/reports/consumer_protection/oft780.pdf, accessed on 12 March 2013.

11. Silversides, A. (2011) 'Long term care in Canada: status quo no option.' The Canadian Federation of Nurses Unions. www.nursesunions.ca/sites/default/files/long_term_care_paper.final__0.pdf, accessed on 31 December 2012.

12. National Union of Public and General Employees (2007) *Dignity Denied: Long-Term Care and Canada's Elderly*. Available at www.nupge.ca/files/images/pdf/Dignity_Denied.pdf, accessed on 31 December 2012.

13. Cranswick, K. and Dosman, D. (2008) 'Eldercare: what we know today.' Available at www.statcan.gc.ca/pub/11-008-x/2008002/article/10689-eng.pdf, accessed on 31 December 2012.

14. Sloane, P.D., Lindeman, D.A., Phillips, C. *et al.* (1995) 'Evaluating Alzheimer's special care units: reviewing the evidence and identifying potential sources of study bias.' The *Gerontologist 35*, 103–111.

15. Sloane, P.D., Lindeman, D.A., Phillips, C. *et al.* (1995) 'Evaluating Alzheimer's special care units: reviewing the evidence and identifying potential sources of study bias.' The *Gerontologist 35*, 103–111.

16. Brodaty, H., Draper, B. and Low, L.-F. (2003) 'Behavioural and psychological symptoms of dementia – a 7 tiered model of service delivery.' *Medical Journal of Australia 178*, 231–234.

17. Australian Institute of Health and Welfare (2009) *Residential Aged Care in Australia 2007-2008: A Statistical Overview. Aged Care Statistic Series 28*. Cat. no. AGE 58. Canberra: AIHW.

18. NHS Choices (undated) 'Community care assessments.' Available at www.nhs.uk/CarersDirect/guide/assessments/Pages/Communitycareassessments.aspx, accessed on 31 December 2012.

19. Care Quality Commission (undated) 'Reports, surveys and reviews.' Available at www.cqc.org.uk/public/reports-surveys-and-reviews, accessed on 31 December 2012.

20. Accreditation Canada (undated) 'Long-term care services.' Available at www.accreditation.ca/accreditation-programs/qmentum/standards/long-term-care-services/, accessed on 31 December 2012.

21. Silversides, A. (2011) 'Long term care in Canada: status quo no option.' The Canadian Federation of Nurses Unions. www.nursesunions.ca/sites/default/files/long_term_care_paper.final__0.pdf, accessed on 31 December 2012.

22. National Union of Public and General Employees (2007) *Dignity Denied: Long-Term Care and Canada's Elderly*. Available at www.nupge.ca/files/images/pdf/Dignity_Denied.pdf, accessed on 31 December 2012.

23. US Department of Health and Human Services (2011) *Your Guide to Choosing a Nursing Home*. Available at www.medicare.gov/Pubs/pdf/02174.pdf, accessed on 31 December 2012.

24. Department of Health and Ageing (2008) *Report to the Minister for Ageing on Residential Care and People with Psychogeriatric Disorders*. Available at: www.health.gov.au/internet/main/publishing.nsf/Content/ageing-quality-report-psychogeriatric-disorders.htm, accessed 1 April 2013.

25. Australian Institute of Health and Welfare (2009) *Residential Aged Care in Australia 2007–2008: A Statistical Overview. Aged Care Statistic Series 28*. Cat. no. AGE 58. Canberra: AIHW.

26. Jeon, Y.H. (2012) 'Psychogeriatric nursing workforce in Australia: an endangered species?' Available at www.ipa-online.org/ipaonlinev4/main/homepagearticles/pnwa.html, accessed on 31 December 2012.

27. Productivity Commission (2011) *Caring for Older Australians: Overview*. Report No. 53, Final Inquiry Report. Canberra: Productivity Commission.

Chapter 12

1. Perkins, C.J. (2001) 'Ethical Issues in Geriatric Psychiatry Liaison.' In P. Melding and B. Draper (eds) *Geriatric Consultation Liaison Psychiatry.* Oxford: Oxford University Press.

2. O'Neill, N. and Peisah, C. (2012) *Capacity and the Law.* Sydney: Sydney University Press.

3. Darzins, P., Molloy, D.W. and Strang, D. (eds) (2000) *Who Can Decide? The Six Step Capacity Assessment Process.* Adelaide: Memory Australia Press.

4. Guardianship Tribunal (undated) Information sheets. Available at www.gt.nsw.gov.au/gt/gt_sheets.html, accessed on 31 December 2012.

5. Reamy, A.M., Kim, K., Zarit, S. and Whitlach, C. (2011) 'Understanding discrepancy in perceptions of values: individuals with mild to moderate dementia and their family caregivers.' The Gerontologist 51, 4, 473–483. doi: 10.1093/geront/gnr010.

6. Reamy, A.M., Kim, K., Zarit, S. and Whitlach, C. (2013) 'Values and preferences of individuals with dementia: perceptions of family caregivers over time.' *The Gerontologist 53,* 2, 293–302.doi: 10.1093/geront/gns078\.

7. Menne, H.L and Whitlach, C. (2007) 'Decision-making involvement of individuals with dementia.' The Gerontologist 47, 6, 810–819. doi: 10.1093/geront/47.6.810.

8. Alzheimer Scotland (2012) 'Dementia: making decisions.' Available at: http://dementiascotland.org/news/files/Dementia-Making-Decisions.pdf, accessed on 1 April 2013.

9. O'Neill, N. and Peisah, C. (2012) *Capacity and the Law.* Sydney: Sydney University Press.

10. Gov.UK. 'Lasting power of attorney.' Available at: www.gov.uk/power-of-attorney/overview, accessed on 1 April 2013.

11. O'Neill, N. and Peisah, C. (2012) *Capacity and the Law.* Sydney: Sydney University Press.

12. Darzins, P., Molloy, D.W. and Strang, D. (eds) (2000) *Who Can Decide? The Six Step Capacity Assessment Process.* Adelaide: Memory Australia Press.

13. O'Neill, N. and Peisah, C. (2012) *Capacity and the Law.* Sydney: Sydney University Press.

14. Darzins, P., Molloy, D.W. and Strang, D. (eds) (2000) *Who Can Decide? The Six Step Capacity Assessment Process.* Adelaide: Memory Australia Press.

15. Guardianship Tribunal (undated) Information sheets. Available at www.gt.nsw.gov.au/gt/gt_sheets.html, accessed on 31 December 2012.

16. Dubinsky, R.M., Stein, A.C. and Lyons, K. (2000) 'Practice parameter: risk of driving and Alzheimer's disease (an evidence based review).' Report of the Quality Standards Subcommittee of the American Academy of Neurology. *Neurology 54,* 2205–2211.

17. Hunt, L.A., Murphy, C.F., Carr, D. *et al.* (1997) 'Reliability of the Washington University Road Test: a performance-based assessment for drivers with dementia of the Alzheimer type.' *Archives of Neurology 54,* 6, 707–712.

18. Carr, D.B., Duchek, J. and Morris, J.C. (2000) 'Characteristics of motor vehicle crashes of drivers with dementia of the Alzheimer type.' *Journal of the American Geriatrics Society 48,* 1, 18–22.

19. Appelbaum, P.S. (2002) 'Involving decisionally impaired subjects in research.' American *Journal of Geriatric Psychiatry 10,* 120–124.

20. Fisk, J., Beattie, B. and Donnelly, M. (2007) 'Ethical considerations for decision making for treatment and research participation.' *Alzheimer's and Dementia 3,* 411–417.

21. Stocking, C.B., Hougham, G.W. and Danner, D.D. *et al.* (2007) 'Empirical assessment of a research advance directive for persons with dementia and their proxies.' *Journal of the American Geriatrics Society 55,* 1609–1612.

22. Hughes, J.C. and Louw, S.J. (2002) 'Electronic tagging of people with dementia who wander.' *British Medical Journal 325,* 847.

23. Hertogh, C.M.P.M. and Ribbe, M.W. (1996) 'Ethical aspects of medical decision-making in demented patients: a report from the Netherlands.' *Alzheimer's Disease and Associated Disorders 10*, 11–19.

24. Lambourne, P. and Lambourne, A. (2001) 'Do not resuscitate policies – what do staff and relatives want for patients with severe dementia?' *International Journal of Geriatric Psychiatry 16*, 1107–1109.

25. Cartwright, C.M. and Steinberg, M.A. (2000) 'PEG feeding, dementia and the need for policies and guidelines.' *Australasian Journal on Ageing 19*, 1061–07.

Chapter 13

1.   Henry, M.S., Passmore, A.P. and Todd, S. (*et al.*) (2012) 'The development of effective biomarkers for Alzheimer's disease: a review.' *International Journal of Geriatric Psychiatry.* DOI: 10.1002/gps.3829.

2.   Hampel, H., Broich, K., Hoessler, Y. and Pantel, J. (2009) 'Biological markers for early detection and pharmacological treatment of Alzheimer's disease.' *Dialogues in Clinical Neuroscience 11*, 141–157.

3.   Henry, M.S., Passmore, A.P. and Todd, S. (*et al.*) (2012) 'The development of effective biomarkers for Alzheimer's disease: a review.' *International Journal of Geriatric Psychiatry.* DOI: 10.1002/gps.3829.

4.   Hampel, H., Broich, K., Hoessler, Y. and Pantel, J. (2009) 'Biological markers for early detection and pharmacological treatment of Alzheimer's disease.' *Dialogues in Clinical Neuroscience 11*, 141–157.

5.   Henry, M.S., Passmore, A.P. and Todd, S. (*et al.*) (2012) 'The development of effective biomarkers for Alzheimer's disease: a review.' *International Journal of Geriatric Psychiatry.* DOI: 10.1002/gps.3829.

6.   Henry, M.S., Passmore, A.P. and Todd, S. (*et al.*) (2012) 'The development of effective biomarkers for Alzheimer's disease: a review.' *International Journal of Geriatric Psychiatry.* DOI: 10.1002/gps.3829.

7.   Hampel, H., Broich, K., Hoessler, Y. and Pantel, J. (2009) 'Biological markers for early detection and pharmacological treatment of Alzheimer's disease.' *Dialogues in Clinical Neuroscience 11*, 141–157.

8.   Henry, M.S., Passmore, A.P. and Todd, S. (*et al.*) (2012) 'The development of effective biomarkers for Alzheimer's disease: a review.' *International Journal of Geriatric Psychiatry.* DOI: 10.1002/gps.3829.

9.   Hampel, H., Broich, K., Hoessler, Y. and Pantel, J. (2009) 'Biological markers for early detection and pharmacological treatment of Alzheimer's disease.' *Dialogues in Clinical Neuroscience 11*, 141–157.

10. Henry, M.S., Passmore, A.P. and Todd, S. (*et al.*) (2012) 'The development of effective biomarkers for Alzheimer's disease: a review.' International Journal of Geriatric Psychiatry. DOI: 10.1002/gps.3829.

11. Hampel, H., Broich, K., Hoessler, Y. and Pantel, J. (2009) 'Biological markers for early detection and pharmacological treatment of Alzheimer's disease.' *Dialogues in Clinical Neuroscience 11*, 141–157.

12. ClinicalTrials.gov (undated) Alzheimer's Disease Neuroimaging Initiative 2. http://clinicaltrials.gov/ct2/show/NCT01231971, accessed on 31 December 2012.

13. Henry, M.S., Passmore, A.P. and Todd, S. (*et al.*) (2012) 'The development of effective biomarkers for Alzheimer's disease: a review.' *International Journal of Geriatric Psychiatry.* DOI: 10.1002/gps.3829.

14. Henry, M.S., Passmore, A.P. and Todd, S. (*et al.*) (2012) 'The development of effective biomarkers for Alzheimer's disease: a review.' *International Journal of Geriatric Psychiatry.* DOI: 10.1002/gps.3829.

15. Henry, M.S., Passmore, A.P. and Todd, S. (*et al.*) (2012) 'The development of effective biomarkers for Alzheimer's disease: a review.' *International Journal of Geriatric Psychiatry.* DOI: 10.1002/gps.3829.

16. Henry, M.S., Passmore, A.P. and Todd, S. (*et al.*) (2012) 'The development of effective biomarkers for Alzheimer's disease: a review.' *International Journal of Geriatric Psychiatry.* DOI: 10.1002/gps.3829.

17. Chen, Y., Wolk, D.A., Reddin, J.S. *et al.* (2011) 'Voxel-level comparison of arterial spin-labeled perfusion MRI and FDG-PET in Alzheimer disease.' *Neurology.* WNL.0b013e31823a0ef7; published ahead of print November 16 2011.

18. Henry, M.S., Passmore, A.P. and Todd, S. (*et al.*) (2012) 'The development of effective biomarkers for Alzheimer's disease: a review.' *International Journal of Geriatric Psychiatry.* DOI: 10.1002/gps.3829.

19. CogState: www.cogstate.com, accessed on 31 December 2012.

20. Sperling, R.A., Aisen, P.S., Beckett, L.A. *et al.* (2011) 'Toward defining the preclinical stages of Alzheimer's disease: recommendations from the National Institute on Aging and the Alzheimer's Association workgroup.' *Alzheimer's & Dementia 7*, 280–292.

21. Sun, G.H., Raji, C.A., MacEachern, M.P. and Burke, J.F. (2012) 'Olfactory identification testing as a predictor of the development of Alzheimer's dementia: a systematic review.' *The Laryngoscope 122*, 7, 1455–1462.

22. Sperling, R.A., Aisen, P.S., Beckett, L.A. *et al.* (2011) 'Toward defining the preclinical stages of Alzheimer's disease: recommendations from the National Institute on Aging and the Alzheimer's Association workgroup.' *Alzheimer's & Dementia 7*, 280–292.

23. McKhann, G.M., Knopman, D.S., Chertkow, H. *et al.* (2011) 'The diagnosis of dementia due to Alzheimer's disease: recommendations from the National Institute on Aging–Alzheimer's Association workgroups on diagnostic guidelines for Alzheimer's disease.' *Alzheimer's & Dementia 7*, 263–269.

24. Siberski, J. (2012) 'Dementia and DSM-5: changes, cost, and confusion.' *Aging Well 5*, 6, 12–16.

25. Siberski, J. (2012) 'Dementia and DSM-5: changes, cost, and confusion.' *Aging Well 5*, 6, 12–16.

26. Siberski, J. (2012) 'Dementia and DSM-5: changes, cost, and confusion.' *Aging Well 5*, 6, 12–16.

27. Woodward, M. (2012) 'Drug treatments in development for Alzheimer's disease.' *Journal of Pharmacy Practice and Research 42*, 58–65.

28. Woodward, M. (2012) 'Drug treatments in development for Alzheimer's disease.' *Journal of Pharmacy Practice and Research 42*, 58–65.

29. Piau, A., Nourhashemi, F., Hein, C. *et al.* (2011) 'Progress in the development of new drugs in Alzheimer's disease.' *The Journal of Nutrition, Health & Aging 15*, 45–57.

30. Woodward, M. (2012) 'Drug treatments in development for Alzheimer's disease.' *Journal of Pharmacy Practice and Research 42*, 58–65.

31. Piau, A., Nourhashemi, F., Hein, C. *et al.* (2011) 'Progress in the development of new drugs in Alzheimer's disease.' *The Journal of Nutrition, Health & Aging 15*, 45–57.

32. Tong, G., Wang, J.S., Sverdlov, O. *et al.* (2012) 'Multicenter, randomized, double-blind, placebo-controlled, single-ascending dose study of the oral γ-secretase inhibitor BMS-708163 (Avagacestat): tolerability profile, pharmacokinetic parameters, and pharmacodynamic markers.' *Clinical Therapeutics 34*, 3, 654–667. doi: 10.1016/j.clinthera.2012.01.022.

33. Alzheimer Research Forum (2012) 'Merck Launches Largest Trial of BACE Inhibitor in AD.' Available at www.alzforum.org/new/detail.asp?id=3339, accessed on 31 December 2012.

34. Clinicaltrials.Gov. 'Study of LY2886721 in Mild Cognitive Impairment Due to Alzheimer's Disease or Mild Alzheimer's Disease.' Available at http://clinicaltrials.gov/show/NCT01561430, accessed on 31 December 2012.

35. Woodward, M. (2012) 'Drug treatments in development for Alzheimer's disease.' *Journal of Pharmacy Practice and Research 42*, 58–65.

36. 36. Piau, A., Nourhashemi, F., Hein, C. *et al.* (2011) 'Progress in the development of new drugs in Alzheimer's disease.' *The Journal of Nutrition, Health & Aging 15*, 45–57.

37. Winblad, B., Andreasen, N., Minthon, L. et al. (2012) 'Safety, tolerability, and antibody response of active Aβ immunotherapy with CAD106 in patients with Alzheimer's disease: randomised, double-blind, placebo-controlled, first-in-human study.' Lancet Neurology 11, 7 (July), 597–604. doi: 10.1016/S1474-4422(12)70140-0. Epub 6 June 2012.

38. Woodward, M. (2012) 'Drug treatments in development for Alzheimer's disease.' *Journal of Pharmacy Practice and Research 42*, 58–65.

39. Piau, A., Nourhashemi, F., Hein, C. *et al.* (2011) 'Progress in the development of new drugs in Alzheimer's disease.' *The Journal of Nutrition, Health & Aging 15*, 45–57.

40. Woodward, M. (2012) 'Drug treatments in development for Alzheimer's disease.' *Journal of Pharmacy Practice and Research 42*, 58–65.

41. Piau, A., Nourhashemi, F., Hein, C. *et al.* (2011) 'Progress in the development of new drugs in Alzheimer's disease.' *The Journal of Nutrition, Health & Aging 15*, 45–57.

42. Alzheimer Research Forum (2012) 'DIAN trial picks Gantenerumab, Solanezumab, maybe BACE inhibitor.' Available at www.alzforum.org/new/detail.asp?id=3289, accessed on 31 December 2012.

43. Sabbagh, M.N. (2009) 'Drug development for Alzheimer's disease: where are we now and where are we headed?' *The American Journal of Geriatric Pharmacotherapy 7*, 167–185.

44. Alzheimer's Society (2012) 'Stem Cell Research.' www.alzheimers.org.uk/site/scripts/documents_info.php?documentID=1039, accessed on 31 December 2012.

45. Galvin, K.A. and Jones, D.G. (2002) 'Adult human neural stem cells for cell-replacement therapies in the central nervous system.' *Medical Journal of Australia 177*, 316–318.

46. Woodward, M. (2012) 'Drug treatments in development for Alzheimer's disease.' *Journal of Pharmacy Practice and Research 42*, 58–65.

47. Piau, A., Nourhashemi, F., Hein, C. et al. (2011) 'Progress in the development of new drugs in Alzheimer's disease.' *The Journal of Nutrition, Health & Aging 15*, 45–57.

48. Tong, G., Wang, J.S., Sverdlov, O. et al. (2012) 'Multicenter, randomized, doubleblind, placebo-controlled, single-ascending dose study of the oral γ-secretase inhibitor BMS-708163 (Avagacestat): tolerability profile, pharmacokinetic parameters, and pharmacodynamic markers.' *Clinical Therapeutics 34*, 3, 654–667. doi: 10.1016/j.clinthera.2012.01.022.

49. Alzheimer Research Forum (2012) 'Merck Launches Largest Trial of BACE Inhibitor in AD.' Available at www.alzforum.org/new/detail.asp?id=3339, accessed on 31 December 2012.

50. Clinicaltrials.Gov. 'Study of LY2886721 in Mild Cognitive Impairment Due to Alzheimer's Disease or Mild Alzheimer's Disease.' Available at: http://clinicaltrials.gov/show/NCT01561430, accessed on 31 December 2012.

51. Alzheimer Research Forum (2012) 'DIAN trial picks Gantenerumab, Solanezumab, maybe BACE inhibitor.' Available at www.alzforum.org/new/detail.asp?id=3289, accessed on 31 December 2012.

52. Sabbagh, M.N. (2009) 'Drug development for Alzheimer's disease: where are we now and where are we headed?' *The American Journal of Geriatric Pharmacotherapy 7*, 167–185.

53. Bharucha, A.J., Anand, V., Forlizzi, J. *et al.* (2009) 'Intelligent assistive technology applications to dementia care: current capabilities, limitations, and future challenges.' *American Journal of Geriatric Psychiatry 17*, 88–104.

54. Crete-Nishihata, M., Baecker, R.M., Massimi, M. *et al.* (2012) 'Reconstructing the past: personal memory technologies are not just personal and not just for memory.' *Human–Computer Interaction 27*, 92–123.

55. Bharucha, A.J., Anand, V., Forlizzi, J. *et al.* (2009) 'Intelligent assistive technology applications to dementia care: current capabilities, limitations, and future challenges.' *American Journal of Geriatric Psychiatry 17*, 88–104.

56. Sposaro, F., Danielson, J., Tyson, G. (2010) 'iWander: an Android application for dementia patients.' Conf Proc IEEE Eng Med Biol Soc 2010, 3875–3878.

57. Bharucha, A.J., Anand, V., Forlizzi, J. *et al.* (2009) 'Intelligent assistive technology applications to dementia care: current capabilities, limitations, and future challenges.' *American Journal of Geriatric Psychiatry 17*, 88–104.

58. Bharucha, A.J., Anand, V., Forlizzi, J. *et al.* (2009) 'Intelligent assistive technology applications to dementia care: current capabilities, limitations, and future challenges.' *American Journal of Geriatric Psychiatry 17*, 88–104.

59. Alzheimer's Disease International (2009) *World Alzheimer Report 2009.* Edited by M. Prince and J. Jackson. Available at www.alz.co.uk/research/world-report, accessed on 8 December 2012.

60. Weon, B.M. and Je, J.H. (2009) 'Theoretical estimation of maximum human lifespan.' Biogerontology 10, 1 (Feb), 65–71. doi: 10.1007/s10522-008-9156-4. Epub 17 June 2008.

61. Economics Help. 'Dependency ratio.' Available at: www.economicshelp.org/dictionary/d/dependency-ratio.html, accessed on 1 April 2013.

Index